COVID-19 AND SHAME

Critical Interventions in the Medical and Health Humanities

Series Editors
Stuart Murray, Corinne Saunders, Sowon Park and Angela Woods

Critical Interventions in the Medical and Health Humanities promotes a broad range of scholarly work across the Medical and Health Humanities, including both larger-scale intellectual projects and argument-led provocations, to present new field-defining, interdisciplinary research into health and human experience.

COVID-19 AND SHAME

POLITICAL EMOTIONS AND PUBLIC HEALTH IN THE UK

Fred Cooper, Luna Dolezal and Arthur Rose

BLOOMSBURY ACADEMIC
LONDON • NEW YORK • OXFORD • NEW DELHI • SYDNEY

BLOOMSBURY ACADEMIC
Bloomsbury Publishing Plc
50 Bedford Square, London, WC1B 3DP, UK
1385 Broadway, New York, NY 10018, USA
29 Earlsfort Terrace, Dublin 2, Ireland

BLOOMSBURY, BLOOMSBURY ACADEMIC and the Diana logo are
trademarks of Bloomsbury Publishing Plc

First published in Great Britain 2023
Reprinted 2023

A catalogue record for this book is available from the British Library.

A catalog record for this book is available from the Library of Congress.
Names: Cooper, Fred (Historian of medicine), author. | Dolezal,
Luna, author. | Rose, Arthur, 1981- author.
Title: COVID-19 and shame : political emotions and public health in the
UK / Fred Cooper, Luna Dolezal and Arthur Rose.
Description: London, UK ; New York, NY, USA :
Bloomsbury Academic/Bloomsbury Publishing Plc, 2023. |
Series: Critical interventions in the medical and health humanities |
Summary: "This open access book examines the various ways that shame and stigma became an
integral part of the United Kingdom's public health response to COVID-19 during 2020, this book argues
that there is an urgent need for public health interventions that are "shame sensitive," addressing
the experience of shame as a crucial, if often overlooked, consequence of such interventions. As the
Covid-19 pandemic unfolded in 2020, interventions by the UK government maximised rather than
minimized experiences of shame and stigma. From healthcare workers insulted in the streets to the
online shaming of "Covidiots" and the "lepers of Leiceister," for example, public animus about the
pandemic found scapegoats for its frustrations. But, rather than intervene with robust strategies to
sensitize people about the effects of this behaviour, the government's healthcare policies and rhetoric
seemed to exacerbate experiences of shame and stigma, relying on a language that intensified
oppositional, antagonistic thinking, while dissimulating about its own responsibilities. Through a series
of case studies around topics such as 'fat shaming', the term 'covidiots', and racial profiling, this
provocative book identifies a systemic failure to manage stigma and shame-producing circumstances in
four key 'scenes': healthcare contexts, social situations, domestic life and political decision-making. The
open access edition of this book is available under a CC BY 4.0 licence on www.bloomsburycollections.
com. Open access was funded by The Wellcome Trust"– Provided by publisher.
Identifiers: LCCN 2022031213 | ISBN 9781350283404 (PB) | ISBN 9781350283411
(HB) | ISBN 9781350283428 (ePDF) | ISBN 9781350283435 (eBook)
| ISBN 9781350283442
Subjects: LCSH: COVID-19 (Disease)–Social aspects. |
COVID-19 Pandemic, 2020–Great Britain–Social aspects. | Shame.
Classification: LCC RA644.C67 C663 2023 |
DDC 362.1962/4144–dc23/eng/20221003
LC record available at https://lccn.loc.gov/2022031213

ISBN: HB: 978-1-3502-8341-1
            PB: 978-1-3502-8340-4
            ePDF: 978-1-3502-8342-8
            eBook: 978-1-3502-8343-5

Series: Critical Interventions in the Medical and Health Humanities

Typeset by Integra Software Services Pvt. Ltd.
Printed and bound in Great Britain

To find out more about our authors and books visit www.bloomsbury.com
and sign up for our newsletters.

CONTENTS

ACKNOWLEDGEMENTS

The research and writing of this book were made possible by the 'Scenes of Shame and Stigma in COVID-19' research grant, funded by the UKRI Arts and Humanities Research Council [AH/V013483/1], and the 'Shame and Medicine' research grant funded by the Wellcome Trust [217879/Z/19/Z]. We would like to thank the Wellcome Trust for enabling us to make this work Open Access; Alice Waterson, who has provided invaluable administrative support and project coordination throughout the research and writing of this book; and the Wellcome Centre for Cultures and Environments of Health (WCCEH) at the University of Exeter, which has provided a supportive transdisciplinary work environment where our research collaboration has thrived. We would also like to thank the Pandemic and Beyond Project for giving us opportunities to share our research and policy recommendations with broader audiences, and the Mass Observation Archive for generous use of their Covid-19 collections. Finally, we would like to thank the editorial team at Bloomsbury Academic and the editors of the series of which this book is a part.

COVID-19 AND SHAME 2020 TIMELINE

December 2019

31 December   A 'pneumonia of unknown cause' reported in Wuhan, Hubei Province, China.

January 2020

1 January   Wuhan market closed.

12 January   First case confirmed outside of China in Thailand.

19 January   First case confirmed in the United States, in Washington State, someone who had returned from Wuhan.

30 January   The first two cases of Covid-19 are confirmed in the UK.

February

3 February   Tow-Arboleda Films' short film 'Coughing While Asian Corona Virus' released.

26 February   First tweet to mention Covidiot.

March

1 March   First use of #covidiot on Twitter.

2 March   UK records first official Covid-19 death.

3 March   Boris Johnson boasts about shaking hands with 'everyone' during a visit to a hospital with confirmed Covid-19 cases. SAGE advises against handshaking.

7 March   GP Chris Higgins publicly shamed by Victorian health minister Jenny Mikakos, and #istandwithchrishiggins appears on Twitter.

12 March   Public Health England stops contact tracing, as infections overwhelm available capacity.

11 March   WHO director Tedros Adhanom Ghebreyesus declares a global pandemic.

13 March   The government's chief scientific advisor Sir Patrick Vallance mentions 'herd immunity' in an interview with Sky News, and this is adopted as an informal public health strategy.

Timeline

14 March	The United States extends its European travel ban to include the UK.
16 March	Boris Johnson advises a halt to nonessential contact and travel; 'Covidiot' appears in *The Urban Dictionary*.
22 March	Columbia Road Flower Market becomes the target of online shaming.
23 March	Boris Johnson announces UK national lockdown ordering people to 'stay at home'.
25 March	The first two NHS doctors die of Covid-19; both are ethnic minorities. Boris Johnson announces a plan to deliver 250,000 tests a day, without a timeline.
26 March	UK lockdown measures legally come into force; the first 'Clap for Carers' tribute takes place with millions applauding NHS and other key workers at 8pm.
27 March	Boris Johnson tests positive for Covid-19; Dominic Cummings drives 250 miles to Durham with his family for 'childcare'.
29 March	The first NHS nurse dies of Covid-19.

April

2 April	Matt Hancock announces plans to carry out 100,000 tests a day by the end of April.
5 April	#selfishpricks hashtag appears on Twitter; Boris Johnson admitted to St Thomas' hospital with Covid-19; Head of State, Elizabeth Windsor, addresses the UK in a special broadcast about Covid-19, and in this broadcast she quotes the Vera Lynn song 'We'll Meet Again'. Belly Mujinga dies at Barnet Hospital having allegedly been spat on by a man who claimed to have the virus.
6 April	Boris Johnson admitted to intensive care.
9 April	A study in Australia finds 61 per cent of doctors feel 'guilt or shame' for wearing a mask because of PPE shortages.
12 April	Boris Johnson is discharged from hospital.
16 April	The Second World War veteran Sir Tom Moore completes 100 laps of his garden, eventually raising £32 million for the NHS Charities Together.
18 April	Executive director of the National Care Forum, Vic Rayner, announces 'a ring of steel' is needed to protect

| | care homes. Comprehensive testing is delivered in September. |
| 22 April | Mumsnet post appears: 'To think I shouldn't be Named and Shamed'. |

May

1 May	Matt Hancock claims to have met the government's testing pledge, with 122,347 tests on 30 April. Experts query the way the government arrives at this figure.
10 May	'Stay Alert' replaces 'Stay at Home' as the UK Government's Guidance. #covidiot surges on Twitter.
11 May	Boris Johnson implores the nation to deploy 'good solid British common sense' in their approach to Covid-19; the UK government advises people to wear facemasks when in indoor spaces such as public transport and shops.
15 May	Boris Johnson attends a party at Downing Street.
20 May	Boris Johnson attends a party at Downing Street.
22 May	Annemarie Plas suggests that the 'Clap for Carers' tribute, which she had originated, should end.
25 May	Dominic Cummings gives a press conference in the Downing Street Rose Garden to defend his trip to Durham and Barnard Castle.
25 May	The murder of George Floyd in Minneapolis, Minnesota.
29 May	Belly Mujinga's case closed with no further action, prompting protests which dovetail with Black Lives Matter demonstrations over the murder of George Floyd.
28 May	The final 'Clap for Carers' tribute.

June

6 June	Anti-racism demonstrations are held across the UK.
18 June	Matt Hancock makes outbreak in Leicester public, gesturing to increasingly local strategy.
19 June	Boris Johnson attends a birthday celebration in the Downing Street Cabinet Room.
24 June	Trump uses the phrase 'Kung Flu' to describe Covid-19 at a rally in Phoenix.

Timeline

24 June	Amnesty report shows the pandemic has led to greater 'marginalisation, stigmatisation and violence' in twelve countries including the UK.
25 June	National news outlets report on huge crowds at Bournemouth beach.
29 June	First 'local lockdown' announced in Leicester and surrounding areas.

July

2 July	Newspaper outlets report a holiday park in Cornwall closing its doors to holidaymakers from Leicester; one resident describes feeling like a 'Leicester Leper'.
4 July	'Local lockdown' in Leicester comes into force; UK 'independence day' with lockdown restrictions lifting in most regions.
24 July	Face coverings become compulsory indoors in England.
25 July	Public Health England publishes a report outlining how being overweight or living with obesity increases the risk of severe illness and death as a result of Covid-19.
27 July	Department of Health and Social Care announces a new 'Tackling Obesity' strategy – 'lose weight to beat COVID-19 and protect NHS'; Number 10 Downing Street release a social media video as part of UK's anti-obesity drive, featuring Boris Johnson stating 'I was too fat' when he was ill with Covid-19.
30 July	Matt Hancock announces heightened restrictions for much of Northern England at short notice on the eve of the Muslim religious holiday Eid al-Adha.

August

3 August	'Eat Out to Help Out' scheme launched to reinvigorate the economy, subsidising prices at restaurants, cafes, and takeaways.
14 August	Lockdown restrictions further eased, particularly in the leisure and culture industries.
31 August	'Selfish covidiots' on a flight from UK to Greek Islands criticized.

September

9 September	Boris Johnson announces the policy known as Operation Moonshot.
10 September	Matt Hancock defends Operation Moonshot in the House of Commons.
14 September	'Rule of Six' imposed, limiting indoor and outdoor meetings to a maximum of six people.
16 September	Boris Johnson appears in the Commons to defend mass testing.
23 September	Boris Johnson returns to the Commons to defend mass testing.
28 September	*The New Yorker* Article 'The Public-Shaming Pandemic' published.

October

2 October	US President Donald Trump tests positive for Covid-19.
6 October	'I was too fat', Boris Johnson explains in reference to the severity of his April Covid-19 illness in his address to the Conservative Party Conference.
14 October	Tier system adopted, allocating medium, high and very high statuses to geographical areas, with a corresponding severity of regulations.
31 October	National lockdown announced.

November

1 November	Testing Capacity exceeds 500,000 tests a day, although only just over 270,000 PCR tests are conducted.
5 November	Second national Lockdown comes into force.
13 November	Two parties take place at Downing Street.

December

2 December	National lockdown ends, with new three-tier system adopted.
8 December	Ninety-year-old Margaret Keenan becomes the first person in the world to receive a Covid-19 vaccine as part of a mass vaccination programme.
15 December	Boris Johnson attends a Downing Street Christmas Quiz.

Timeline

18 December	A party takes place at Downing Street.
19 December	Boris Johnson announces tougher restrictions for London and the South East, with a new tier 4 alert level, 'stay home'.
21 December	UK dubbed 'plague island' in *The New York Times*.
24 December	Brexit deal finalized by Boris Johnson.
25 December	Christmas day, up to three households allowed to mix.
26 December	Tier 4 expanded to encompass more areas of England.
31 December	78 per cent of English population under Tier 4 restrictions.

INTRODUCTION: THE PUBLIC SHAMING PANDEMIC

22 April 2020. The UK's first lockdown. A distressed mother takes to Mumsnet, a London-based forum for parents, to invite support from their popular 'Am I being unreasonable?' thread. 'To think', she begins, 'I shouldn't be named and shamed for not clapping'.[1] 'Clapping', by this point, has become synonymous with a Thursday night ritual, what came to be known as 'Clap for Carers', when those staying at home congregate at their doors to celebrate the work of the UK's National Health Service (NHS) by clapping and banging pots and pans. Ostensibly a positive gesture aimed at boosting the morale of the confined and applauding healthcare and other frontline workers, Clap for Carers had more insidious implications, as the mother realizes:

> I clapped originally and it was lovely and everyone turned out for it here. Last week, after a rough night with DS [dear son] I fell asleep after he went down and missed the clapping. A post went on our community Facebook group actually naming and shaming me. I was mortified. The post said everyone else turned out and I showed the street up and if I can't spend a minute showing my appreciation I don't deserve to use the NHS if I or my family get ill. I ignored it at the time but I can't get it out of my head it's really upset me.[2]

The consensus on the forum was no, she was not being unreasonable. The story had struck a chord. At least a dozen newspapers reported it with headlines such as: 'Exhausted mum "named and shamed" for sleeping through Clap for Carers'.[3] Around the same time, others came forward to report similar experiences about the Thursday night clap. A *Financial Times* article noted: 'Awful stories circulated of people being chastised for missing it, even when the reason was they were NHS shift workers trying to catch up on sleep.'[4] A month later, Clap for Carers would end, skewered by criticisms that it was a 'hollow gesture', co-opted by politicians eager to turn public attention away from the scandalous shortages of Personal Protective Equipment (PPE) that plagued the NHS in the early pandemic.[5]

The Mumsnet post tells the story of a person who has been publicly shamed by a neighbour, outed visibly as falling short of a new collective norm. To redeem herself in her own eyes, she turns to a forum where her neighbour's actions will be judged and found wanting. On its own, the post appears to describe one isolated incident. Put into sequence with other, similar events, it serves as an exemplar of what D. T. Max would later call 'the public-shaming pandemic': the surge in bids to name, blame and shame people by self-appointed guardians of the public good.[6] Like many such instances of what we term pandemic shaming, the story shows how offline actions came to be reproduced online as either reproof or defence, how events, groups and fora meant to build community spirit led to divisions over who was considered morally worthy and unworthy, and how this often happened at the expense of the vulnerable and the marginalized.

As stories such as this began to proliferate during the UK's first lockdown and after, they consolidated a pattern of shame and shaming within the UK's pandemic landscape that seemed, if not directed by an overarching plan, at least symptomatic of a series of recurring missteps. To understand this pattern, this book uses six case studies from 2020 that elucidate the ways that shame and shaming became central to the UK's pandemic experience.

Covid-19 and shame: Contexts

First reported in Wuhan, the capital city of China's Hubei province, in the closing days of 2019, the contagious respiratory illness Covid-19 rapidly spread across the world. Caused by contact with the SARS-CoV-2 strain of coronavirus, largely through airborne transmission from person to person, Covid-19 typically results in symptoms such as coughing, fever, loss of taste and smell, and breathing difficulties. While for some these symptoms are comparatively mild, or even non-existent, for others Covid-19 is a life-threatening disease. It can also have long-term effects on the respiratory and vascular systems. Survivors have frequently reported experiencing something resembling chronic fatigue, a condition now dubbed 'Long Covid'.[7]

For the vast majority in the UK, Covid-19 shifted from looming threat to direct and unavoidable intrusion in March 2020. Although the virus had been circulating for several months, the first UK death was recorded on the 2nd;[8] the World Health Organization (WHO) designated Covid-19 a pandemic on the 11th;[9] and government advice was updated daily, before a full 'lockdown', consisting of considerable quarantine restrictions and characterized by spending twenty-three hours a day at home, came into legal force on the 26th. From early May, these restrictions were gradually relaxed. A new approach was adopted. Geographical tiers and 'local lockdowns' kept some parts of the country in complete or partial quarantine, while others enjoyed a relative return to 'normality'. Close to a third of employees in the UK were furloughed across the spring and summer, with many precarious workers simply losing their jobs. As deaths mounted in the autumn, a two-week 'circuit-breaker' was attempted to avoid harsher restrictions at Christmas. The country was then placed back into quarantine. By the close of 2020, the UK had been dubbed 'Plague Island' by the international community.[10] Covid-19 had been implicated in 72,178 UK deaths, 2,280,658 confirmed cases, extensive disruption, painful and terrifying experiences of acute and chronic illness, and largely unresolved collective grief.[11]

From the outset of the first UK lockdown, it became clear that the material mitigations put in place by the UK government (the Stay at Home order; the furlough scheme) would not provide the necessary scaffolding for responding to the vastly different infrastructural and psychological needs of individuals and communities. Perhaps understandable in the frantic early stages of the pandemic, public health injunctions would continue to collapse a vast range of contexts, experiences and realities into black-and-white imperatives, presupposing homes, resources, relationships and circumstances which made compliance bearable.[12] Even with sustained academic, charitable and activist attention to mental and physical health over the past two years, the vast and complicated nexus of stress, grief, loneliness, estrangement, abandonment, frustration and pain produced by the lockdowns is only beginning to be understood.[13] Shame, we argue, has been an important component of this (primarily individualized) collective suffering, exacerbating and complicating other negative experiences and emotions.

In the UK, as elsewhere, 'pandemic shaming', that is, the public naming, blaming and shaming of individuals and groups, was a widely reported phenomenon during the early stages of the Covid-19 pandemic, especially during lockdowns. Members of the public, often neighbours, policed the behaviour, actions and intentions of others through public censure and opprobrium, often on social media. Stories like the Mumsnet post led, in turn, to media attention, social bemusement and commentary. From April 2020, articles in UK and US news outlets began to reflect on the phenomenon in general, puzzling over its origins and weighing in on shaming as a public health strategy.[14] Many of these looked at the UK's first lockdown, where police were inundated with thousands of complaints and reports about people allegedly breaking lockdown rules, and neighbours were routinely informing on each other. The reasons they gave ranged from not adhering to the rules (such as guests staying overnight, illegal indoor gatherings, rule-breaking excursions) to poor social etiquette (such as hoarding toilet paper or improper hand washing).

Pandemic shaming was enabled by the rapid formation and spread of virtual groups on Facebook and WhatsApp, created by physical neighbours to stay in touch and help each other out during lockdown. Although often started with the noblest of intentions, solidarity and shaming frequently inhabited the same virtual spaces. At times, the groups became mediums for 'curtain twitching', or the unspoken, unofficial surveillance or monitoring of one's neighbours. So-called pandemic 'transgressions', as in the Mumsnet example above, were documented by ordinary citizens on these platforms and elsewhere, presumably looking out for themselves and other concerned members of their community.

For those forced to stay at home, online spaces became sites for airing personal and local grievances that occurred offline and, by extension, helped to circulate shame and censure. Hashtags like #covidiot, a neologism combining covid and idiot, proliferated through the UK Twittersphere as a shorthand for naming, blaming and shaming individuals and groups linked to particular images or stories. But pandemic shaming did not just land on the so-called 'idiots' who ignored or flaunted public health rules. It also became a means to enact a moralizing surveillance on those deemed not to be behaving with pandemic propriety. In this regard, it acquired a ritualistic function: acting both to confirm the need to behave in a particular way and to reinforce the community in whose name these behaviours were demanded.

In the late 1980s, the historian of medicine Charles Rosenberg observed that epidemics are frequently accompanied by such 'collective rites integrating cognitive and emotional elements'.[15] These rites worked simultaneously to affirm belief – in 'religion, in rationalistic pathology, or in some combination of the two' – and to provide reassurance through the familiarity of ritual and the assertion of group identity.[16] They can be traced across different historical epidemics, although their tenor and composition necessarily changes. In the UK in 2020, a series of conditions allowed cynical or careless uses of shame in political and public health discourses to become ritualized in public attitudes, emotions and behaviour. This impetus to shame members of particular groups was not new. But, neither should it simply be read as a 'natural' or 'inevitable' expression of public dismay. Rather, it tells us something important about the contexts in which this impetus occurs.

Direct acts of pandemic shaming in 2020, as illustrated by our Mumsnet example, were not merely random expressions of individual grievances unique to the Covid-19 pandemic. Instead, these visible instances of explicit shaming were surface manifestations of broader patterns of social and political ideologies, policies and power relations. Much of what we discuss in this book is simultaneously very new *and* rooted in deeper processes and pasts, whether militaristic rhetoric about the NHS (Chapter 2), histories of anti-Asian racism (Chapter 3) or the adoption of neoliberal ideologies within public health (Chapter 4). We have largely avoided drawing parallels or 'learning lessons' from histories of epidemiology or societal responses to epidemics, outbreaks and plagues – except when demonstrating lineages of shame.[17] A vibrant field of historical scholarship on past pandemics is in the process of situating Covid-19 within longer temporalities of infectious disease to do just that.[18] Instead, we consider the pandemic events of 2020, in the UK, through a shame lens.

Why shame?

Shame is an emotion that is often central to experiences of illness, infection, contamination and stigmatization. Shame has long been associated with public health, and campaigns frequently mobilize it to motivate 'good', 'proper' or 'healthy' behaviour. Our interest in shame goes far beyond the impact of public health campaigns on individuals. In this work, we deploy shame to make salient a range of *personal emotional experiences*, along with *expressions and experiences of social and political power* which arose in the UK during 2020, as a result of a diverse range of phenomena, including, but not limited to, public health policy, communications, discourse and practice, political rhetoric, mainstream media and socio-cultural narratives. Our discussion of shame highlights some of the intersections between politics, emotions, public health and personal experience.

What is shame? Shame has been called the 'master emotion'[19] and a 'keystone affect',[20] with many philosophers, sociologists and psychologists seeing shame as centrally significant for understanding subjectivity, identity and social relations.[21] Shame is commonly understood to be a personal experience that arises when one feels judged by another or others (whether they are present, imagined or internalized) to have transgressed or broken a social rule or norm. Sociologists such as Erving Goffman have suggested that shame is ubiquitous in our experience, where the threat of shame and embarrassment is the unspoken force that keeps us in line with others and maintains social order.[22] Hence, shame avoidance is woven into the fabric of our human and social relationships; it keeps us in harmony with others, ensuring our physical and social survival. As we learn rules and habits of conduct and behaviour, we become adept at following norms and avoiding shame.

While shame may perform some necessary social functions, too much shame can be compromising, unhealthy, oppressive and potentially 'toxic'.[23] Instead of facilitating personal, moral and social growth, excessive shame can be destructive, leading to a diminished personal and social existence. There is evidence that unhealthy or toxic shame leads to profound disempowerment, lack of political engagement, concrete disadvantage, lack of empathy, the breakdown of social relationships, negative health outcomes, mental ill health, addiction and violence, and is correlated with a wide range of other deleterious social outcomes.[24] In short, while shame serves an important role in human socialization, it can easily become a very negative phenomenon.

Shame is consequently a powerful political emotion. It can be mobilized to manipulate, coerce and motivate others. Often, those with high levels of social power use it for purposes of control, conformity, punishment or exclusion.[25] Preying on cultural concerns regarding belonging, embodied connection, reputation and status, shame, when intentionally exacerbated (by individuals, groups or social structures), can punish, isolate, oppress, disadvantage or marginalize certain individuals, groups or populations. In addition, shame experiences vary according to vulnerability. Some individuals are more shame-prone, meaning that they are more likely to feel shame and be harmed by its negative effects.[26] Shame-proneness is often correlated with negative social experiences such as stigma, trauma, poverty, outsider status, minority status or being lower down the social hierarchy.

An almost universal human motivation to avoid shame, exacerbated by one's relative shame-proneness, means shame can be used to coerce and control people. This can be done through obvious acts of intentional stigmatization or shaming, or more covertly, by manipulating social norms, that is, when those who hold power change rules about what is 'right', 'legal', 'acceptable' or 'moral'.

The contours of shame experiences shifted dramatically during the early stages of the pandemic, when rules, laws and guidance regarding social distancing changed rapidly. For instance, wearing a facemask was initially perceived as an outrageous overreaction, with many people reporting feeling shame and embarrassment wearing masks in public.[27] Initially, mask wearing in the UK was marked by public shaming, ridicule and harassment. This changed as many shops made mask wearing compulsory. The practice shifted from signifying illness to signifying concern over its spread.[28] Eventually, on 23 July 2020, the UK government made mask wearing in indoor settings mandatory. From that date, shame and embarrassment were deemed undeniably appropriate for those who refused to wear a mask indoors.

This example illustrates shame's chameleon-like quality. What is shameful shifts and changes. It is experienced very differently by individuals depending on context, circumstances, personal history, culture and many other factors. One person's shame may scarcely register as mild embarrassment for someone else. Shame takes many forms and manifests in experience in a variety of different ways. It is a personal emotion, intrinsic to social life and social order. But shame must also be understood through expressions and experiences of social and political power. It is necessarily bound up in shared social, cultural and political norms and values. In this book, we are concerned with what Creed et al. have identified as a 'shame nexus', where 'shame' designates a range of experiences and phenomena that incorporates an individual's private emotional experience, explicit acts of shaming that are intended to shore up the norms, morals and concerns of a community or group, and institutional, socio-cultural and political understandings of what constitutes shameful behaviour.[29] Our analysis in this book focuses on three interrelated ways that shame became apparent in the UK during 2020: (1) the explicit use of shame and shaming, (2) the implicit creation of shame and shaming as a by-product of other policies, actions and practices, and (3) shame avoidance as means for reputation management, or 'saving face'.

While we make these conceptual demarcations to identify three specific 'types' of shame, these are interlinked and overlapping. In our Mumsnet example, a member of the public used explicit shaming to condemn and police the behaviour of an individual. This was in turn met by a 'shame backlash' where the individual who weaponized shame in the first instance was in turn shamed in media responses.[30] Underpinning these instances of explicit shaming was an implicit shame dynamic, rooted in the Clap for Carers phenomena and its intertwining of social cohesion and politics. This provided the social processes and power relations required for shame and shaming to emerge.

In April 2020, Clap for Carers had become a national symbol of 'exemplary' pandemic behaviour. Coming out on your doorstep to cheer and clap for key workers was intended as a point of community cohesion and morale building, while also showing an appreciation for the key workers who continued to work, often with considerable risk to their health, while most were locked down at home. However, Clap for Carers almost instantly became bound up in a nationalistic 'blitz spirit' nostalgia of solidarity against a common 'enemy'. Not clapping came to have a deeper symbolic significance, where the possibility for shame and shaming became potent: one was letting down one's street, one's community, one's *entire nation*.

In addition to these dynamics of explicit and implicit shame and shaming, shame avoidance and face saving became particularly fraught for the UK government. The Thursday night Clap for Carers, and related appreciation initiatives, such as Matt Hancock's April 2020 Badge for Carers, became a way for the government to attempt to save face, avoiding shame and reputation damage, by deflecting attention away from PPE shortages, lack of testing, the crisis in care homes, and the poor pay and working conditions of NHS staff. When Clap for Carers was stopped after ten weeks by its founder Annemarie Plas, she claimed that it was getting too 'politicised', co-opted by those in power to cover over structural issues, like low pay and the charges non-UK healthcare staff had to pay to use the NHS: 'We can give them respect but we are not signing the cheque – that falls on another desk.'[31] Unpacking the Mumsnet example demonstrates the complex dynamics captured by what we mean by 'shame' in this book: a nexus that extends from a personal emotion to expressions and experiences of social and political power, from direct experiences of shame to those of shame avoidance.

Shame, stigma and public health

When shame appears as a structural issue of public health discourses and practices, it usually pertains to stigma, the dominant concept used to explain the social burden that often accompanies illness. Stigma is a well-known idea in legal, medical and social scholarship, used to explain why and how certain individuals or groups experience discrimination, marginalization, vilification, judgement, status-loss, unfair treatment, social exclusion and prejudice.[32] In early 2020, stigma regarding Covid-19 was immediately identified as an urgent issue by the NHS, Public Health England (PHE), WHO, Centers for Disease Control and Prevention (CDC) and other health bodies globally.

Stigma is not something that is experienced *directly* (as we might experience the pain or discomfort associated with an illness or the discomfort associated with racism or other forms of discrimination). Instead, stigma is experienced *indirectly* through association with other events or experiences that one has in social, political or healthcare contexts, such as discrimination, labelling, marginalization or prejudice. These sorts of experiences come to be understood *to be the result of the stigma* associated with one's circumstances or condition.[33] To elucidate how stigma is experienced by individuals, the sociologist Graham Scambler considers the first-person experience of stigma. He discusses 'felt stigma' as a way to distinguish how stigma is *experienced* from the social phenomena (such as discrimination, labelling etc.) usually associated with it.[34]

Scambler suggests that 'felt stigma' has two parts: first, 'the *shame* associated with' being reduced to a condition (e.g., 'being mentally ill' or 'being unemployed'), and second, 'the *fear of encountering enacted stigma*',[35] where 'enacted stigma' is synonymous with 'shaming'.[36] This establishes a necessary relation between shame and the experience of stigma. Scambler is not the only person to posit this connection.[37] But, where he keeps the two distinct, many researchers end up using the terms 'shame' and 'stigma' interchangeably, taking for granted a connection between the *emotion* and *experience* of shame and the *social attribute* or *category* of stigma.

Shame and stigma are distinct. Not all shame is related to stigma. Nor was shame identified as a direct concern by the WHO, CDC, PHE or other public health bodies. This omission is not surprising. Since shame is an emotion that is usually associated with personal failing or inadequacy, the emphasis on stigma in public health discourses saves individuals from carrying the burden or blame for the negative attributes associated to their stigmatized condition or circumstances. Moreover, stigma is recognized as a structural and political (rather than individual) problem.[38] However, not recognizing shame as an important part of the public health landscape misses key factors that lead to personal and collective disadvantage, obscuring the affective dimensions of the political machinery that attempts to coerce, control and disadvantage individuals and groups. In no small way, the ambivalence to shame in public health discourse comes from the contested role it often plays in mobilizing campaigns. Far from being an ill to be addressed, it too often appears as a solution to the problem.

To understand why, we need to recall the emphasis on population-level behavioural change in public-facing public health interventions. As focus shifted to chronic rather than infectious disease in the mid-twentieth century, determinants of health such as diet, exercise, smoking and alcohol consumption increasingly came to be framed as decontextualized matters of lifestyle choice. During this liberalization of public health, campaigns mobilized notions of balance and self-discipline to affirm, as Jane Hand puts it, 'the centrality of the self to risk-factor epidemiology … where the individual held new-found power in dictating health outcomes and contributing to chronic disease reduction'.[39] Within the constraints of public health orthodoxies, the key question becomes how to engage different publics in recognizing and absorbing prevailing norms regarding healthy or safe behaviour. Some public health initiatives attempt to educate audiences, for example, on the deleterious effects of practices which might not be widely known. Others set out to bridge the gap between knowledge that something might be 'bad' for individual or collective health and active determination to make positive changes. Frequently, such campaigns aim at creating an emotional commitment to a particular course of action, whether good pandemic citizenship or mental and physical 'self-care'.

Public health initiatives often seek to mobilize shame, but it is also a highly contested and much-criticized outcome. Defences of shame as a tool for leveraging change rest primarily on the argument that it sometimes works; by appealing to an audience's sense of shame around particular behaviours or practices, it has been possible to effect a shift in habits among some of those targeted.[40] However, evidence also shows that campaigns that use shame, blame or stigma to motivate individuals are often counter-productive, compounding or exacerbating negative health outcomes and ill health, especially for groups that are already vulnerable or living with health inequalities. As Robert Walker notes, 'explicit shame is best avoided as its effects are unpredictable'.[41] Reliably predicting how shame will land is often difficult. It is more likely to harm shame-prone communities and individuals, and people with long experiences of public and structural shame. Shaming also runs the risk of hardening unhealthy behaviour and decreasing receptivity to public health advice, as recipients reject shame and lose trust in institutions and experts.[42] Reviewing evidence from global public health campaigns, the medical anthropologists Alexandra Brewis and Amber Wutich conclude: 'Shame in all its forms needs to be removed from the public health tool kit, because it too easily misfires.'[43]

What is striking in the UK government's public health communications strategy during the first wave of the Covid-19 pandemic is the extent that shame and blame were deployed, despite their dubious status. It seems clear that this 'heaping blame on shame' was a 'wilful political strategy', in Graham Scambler's terms.[44] Shaming and blaming individuals helped to deflect attention from the broader systemic failings that had plagued the UK government's pandemic response. These failures came in a multitude of contexts. Poor pandemic preparedness leading up to 2020 meant that infrastructures and established protocols were not in place to respond swiftly and effectively. Hospitals were plagued with shortages in PPE and trained staff. Staff themselves were battling extensive and long-standing burnout. The British prime minister Boris Johnson compounded these problems by refusing to take the pandemic seriously in its early stages, boasting on the 3rd of March about shaking hands with 'everyone' at a hospital with confirmed coronavirus cases, the same day that the government's Scientific Advisory Group for Emergencies (SAGE) advised 'against greetings such as shaking hands and hugging, given existing evidence about the importance of hand hygiene'.[45]

Johnson's government were reluctant to introduce restrictions, initially pursuing a strategy of 'herd immunity' before the projected loss of life was realized to be politically unpalatable to the public.[46] Having built his career on antagonism towards the so-called 'nanny state', deploring 'interference' in everyday life from either the European Union or successive Labour governments between 1997 and 2010, Johnson (and other senior ministers) prevaricated over introducing quarantine measures which were already in place in other European countries. Without advancing an uncritical view of 'lockdowns', which demand vast supportive infrastructures and can be made less isolating without seriously impacting viral outcomes, it seems reasonable to suggest that acting sooner could have helped to buy time and save lives.

UK public health communications implicitly, and often explicitly, blamed and shamed individuals for the prevalence of the virus (through breaking rules or not using their 'common sense') and for the subsequent overburdening of the NHS (by being overweight, for example). Culpability for the spread and severity of the virus was used to demonize certain groups, often those already socially disadvantaged in some way (e.g., immigrant communities, people of colour, individuals living with obesity, low-paid factory workers), to create scapegoats who could shoulder the blame for political failures. Shame over infections, hospitalizations and deaths had to accrue somewhere. In this context, public health policy and messaging did shadow work in directing blame and shame towards the publics it targeted. In so doing, it drew on some of the most harmful traditions and tendencies in its long and ambivalent history.

It also reflected the broader socio-political conditions of the last forty to fifty years. Socially, the neoliberal turn from the 1970s onwards created conditions that name, blame and shame individuals for systemic issues. 'Neoliberalism' emphasizes narratives of personal responsibility at the expense of the welfare state, and, Scambler argues, 'attributions of shame and blame' are central to the successful maintenance of its social order. The reproduction of the status quo, along with its norms, practices and ideologies, depends on 'rooting out the misfits in all their heterogeneity and the variety and severity of the threats they represent'.[47] Issues such as poverty, unemployment, obesity, chronic illness, addiction and other social ills, therefore, are seen as the result of individuals' personal failings, and a lack of hard work and effort, rather than because of structural and social conditions which concretely disadvantage and harm certain individuals in society, perpetuating and entrenching inequality. Under the logics of neoliberalism this renders 'people personally responsible for their "problems," whatever form these might take'.[48]

In the UK, shaming and blaming individuals for social ills has become a commonplace logic, a neoliberal common sense estranging uncompetitive 'actions' and 'choices' from systems and contexts, and must be seen to have consequences, including for health and social standing.[49] What this 'common sense' often elides, argues Imogen Tyler, are 'the ways in which stigma is purposefully crafted as a strategy of government, in ways that often deliberately seek to foment and accentuate inequalities and injustices'.[50] Although Tyler focuses on stigma, her detailed and rewarding analysis is often concerned with its affective consequences. As she notes: 'when people use the term "stigma" today, they… use it… to describe the debilitating psychological effects of being stigmatised, with a particular emphasis on how the shame induced by stigma corrodes well-being and damages your sense of self'.[51] From austerity to *Benefits Street*, the 'welfare stigma machine', as Tyler calls it, 'tutored the public to believe that people living in poverty were lazy or feckless, and that the forms of distress [it caused] were deserved – a consequence of people's own poor behaviours, bad choices and indiscipline'.[52] In other words, it internalized a particularly pernicious form of shame.

These longer narratives of shame, blame and stigma were invested with new invective in the wake of the major populist events in 2016 (most notably the Brexit Referendum in the UK and the election of Donald Trump as the US president). These events were populist, insofar as they were marked by narratives that structured politics as a fundamental antagonism between 'elites' and 'the people'. In promising to return the UK and the USA to an imagined state of prior greatness, the campaigns headed by Boris Johnson and Donald Trump also represented their respective nations as in a state of humiliation. As Alexandra Homolar and Georg Löfflmann have argued, their narratives emphasized the humiliation of an abandoned 'true people', in order 'to claim experiences of trauma and loss for their audiences, thus fuelling rather than quenching their sense of entitlement and status'.[53] Humiliation narratives have 'a dyadic ability … to affectively anchor populist messaging in feelings of pride and hope on the one hand and anxiety and anger on the other'.[54] When Brexit and Trump voters were routinely called 'idiots', these everyday humiliations supported the overall narrative of these movements, that such supporters were the victims of efforts to control and disempower them. Voting for Brexit and electing Trump became the means to reassert a national pride, a way of redirecting the shame generated by this humiliation.

These contexts, as well as the more immediate context of veiled or overt incitements to shame, created a public animus which contributed to the burden of shame. It is important to stress – particularly in regard to moments we discuss public complicity in shame where – that shame is inextricable from the broader question of power relations. Shaming others can be understood as a (flawed) means of exerting control over situations and circumstances when people feel powerless. With few avenues for restitution for vast collective losses, whether from a virus which cannot be held to account or from a government which rarely seems to be, the fear and frustration which frequently frame attempts to shame are understandable and forgivable emotions. Our critique of shame as a political emotion is not intended, therefore, to shame those who have shamed others; we reproduce these testimonies as a way of demonstrating how 'ordinary' people can be conscripted into the machinery of shame, often acting against their own interests.[55]

Our methods

We write this book as medical humanities scholars from the disciplines of history, philosophy, and literary and cultural studies. A government emphasis on 'following the science' during the pandemic has often marginalized humanities research. This fits a longer pattern of (frequently explicit) devaluation.[56] Nevertheless, work in the humanities is of vital importance to the pandemic, not least because questions of context, communication, experience, emotion, culture and meaning have been – and continue to be – decisive factors in public health, epidemiology and everyday life. The many failures in government policy in the UK in the last two years bear witness to a series of endemic cultural problems, with criticism rife that policymakers did not sufficiently 'follow the science', or that they were sometimes guilty of following the wrong science, e.g., in pursuing eugenic goals of 'herd immunity'. These criticisms sidestep the thornier problem that the sciences alone, even (or perhaps particularly) if 'followed' to the letter, may not value or create the kinds of outcomes cognisant of different forms of social, cultural, and emotional survival or living well.[57] Without a substantial – and genuinely receptive – engagement with the humanities, policymakers will continue to ask the wrong questions and look for answers in the wrong places. This book stands as an example of what collaborative and interdisciplinary humanities scholarship can do, illuminating a host of instances where careful attention to problems and questions central to humanities practice could have made for better policy and resulted in better health.

In tracing the permutations of shame in the first year of the Covid-19 pandemic, we have drawn from diverse sources, including academic research, news stories, policy documents, cultural texts and social media posts. Although this is not a book (primarily) about experience, we have also made extensive use of written testimony, to show how the stories we tell about shame have landed in everyday life. Our analysis moves, therefore, between macroscopic narratives and processes about shame's causes and conditions and microscopic accounts of shame in the thoughts and feelings of real people. Many of the testimonies we explore are taken from the Mass Observation Archive at the University of Sussex. Founded in 1937 by the anthropologist Tom Harrisson, the artist and film-maker Humphrey Jennings and the journalist and poet Charles Madge, Mass Observation set out to record an 'anthropology of ourselves' through a national panel of volunteer writers on ordinary life.[58] The project invites 'mass observers' to respond to focused directives (a set of questions on a particular theme or series of themes, intended to offer a loose structure), and to take detailed diaries for specific days of the year: sometimes random, sometimes corresponding to momentous national and international events. Recent directives and day-diaries reflect a preoccupation with Covid-19 among both respondents and commissioners, with contributions invited from people not usually involved in the Mass Observation project. The archive therefore offers an exceptionally rich resource for the study of experiences, opinions and emotions during the pandemic.

This book takes a case study approach. Each of the six chapters is an in-depth, multi-faceted and multidisciplinary exploration of a complex issue.[59] They demonstrate that a lack of consideration of shame, and its effects and consequences, caused significant harm, and that this harm could *and should* have been avoided. Rather than a comprehensive account of 2020, the book sketches a landscape of political emotions to understand how public health policies were shaped and how many social harms were normalized. Instead of a complete picture of the year and the complex systems and processes at play in the pandemic, we use a 'shame lens' to understand its public health landscape.[60] This provides an important framework for considering the direct and indirect social harms that can result from interventions ostensibly designed to protect individuals and keep populations healthy and safe.

Our chapters

Our six case studies address three interlocking and interconnected strands: (1) the explicit use of shame and shaming, (2) the implicit use of shame and shaming, or in other words, shame as a by-product of interventions and (3) shame avoidance as a means for reputation management, or 'saving face'.

In our first chapter, 'Covidiots!: The language of pandemic shaming', we use a linguistic case study – the formation, use and meaning of the neologism 'covidiot' – to think critically about blame, shame, power and language. From a public means of holding the powerful to account, at least rhetorically, covidiot soon became a way to brand individuals as stupid, selfish, inconsiderate and potentially dangerous. As a method for casting shame, it translated across social media and online and print journalism, collapsing complicated histories and circumstances into simplistic judgements on the intellect and character of the offending party. As an early – and persistent – iteration of pandemic shaming, covidiot created fertile grounds for more and less specific patterns of shame, as individuals were held accountable for complex and contextually embedded behaviours.

Our second chapter, 'Super-spreaders: Shaming healthcare professionals', focuses on an early target for shame: healthcare workers. While the fiction persisted that most infectious cases were receiving medical treatment or located in hospitals, healthcare workers were identified – sometimes personally – as vectors for disease. Discussing a series of high-visibility cases, we situate attempts to publicly shame doctors in longer histories of shame and mistrust during epidemics. Even as healthcare workers were shamed for their proximity to the sick, many were also shamed for their reluctance to work without complaint in dangerous conditions. Underwritten by a nationalistic rhetoric of wartime sacrifice, narratives of heroism, as we explore in this chapter, created fertile ground for shame, blame and stigma.

Discussing the role of shame in racism, our third chapter, 'Coughing While Asian: Shame and Racialized Bodies', considers how members of racialized communities were shamed for their imagined role in the transmission of disease, in ways that followed distinct historical and cultural scripts. Instances of violence, hatred and vitriol towards people (often wrongly) identified as Chinese sought to shame victims as complicit in the spread of the virus, whether through poor hygiene and distasteful eating habits or as part of a longer adversarial dynamic between China and the Global West. Simultaneously, as a disproportionate number of Covid-19 casualties were identified as ethnic minorities, speculation lingered on living arrangements which fell outside of 'white normal', alongside racialized anxieties over public health non-compliance and the use of public space. Through the government policy of 'local lockdowns', large areas, and sometimes entire cities (such as Leicester) were marked with shame, with real social, emotional and relational consequences for inhabitants. These shamed spaces and places tended to have high proportions of racialized communities, and have ongoing histories of underinvestment, abandonment, and stigma. The real reasons for disparities in Covid-19 mortality and morbidity – in short, systemic social and health inequalities caused and determined by endemic racism – relied on and perpetuated shame.

In our fourth chapter, 'I was too fat: Boris Johnson and the fat panic', we address parallel questions over obesity and shame, as government and public health rhetoric placed fresh emphasis on 'simple' lifestyle choices as a way of reducing excess weight, and consequently alleviating pressure on the NHS. Following a long tradition of holding fat bodies accountable for deep-seated structural problems, these discourses collapsed complex challenges into good and bad individual decisions, neither acknowledging nor addressing the multifarious contexts, cultures, histories, relationships, environments and resources involved in making them. With these vital considerations stripped away, those targeted by public health interventions were invested with direct and individual responsibility for managing their weight, their health, and the ability of health systems to cope with the pandemic.

Government rhetoric on 'common sense' held members of the public further accountable for poor pandemic outcomes. In Chapter 5, 'Good Solid British Common Sense: Shame and surveillance in everyday life', we dissect common sense as both popular notion and public health advice. In asking publics to apply common sense, politicians deflected shame from their own handling of the pandemic, invoking individual responsibility and behaviour as a tactic for saving face. Intended to prompt self-surveillance by encouraging the 'use' of common sense, this also became an injunction to judge – and, frequently, to shame – the common sense of others. Making use of testimonies in the Mass Observation Archive which reckon with experiences of shame during the pandemic, we find people who felt their common sense called into question, or surveilled or policed by others. These individuals interpreted rhetorics of common sense and applied them to their own and others' behaviour. In lieu of clear public health messaging, accountability to common sense imposed unnecessary patterns of shaming and shame, in service to a mutable idea with little practical application as a theory of behaviour, but with significant ideological and political consequences.

Finally, our sixth chapter, 'Operation Moonshot: Notes on saving face', develops and unravels the notion of 'saving face', which we use to think about how and why the UK government sought to deflect shame away from themselves with such predictable frequency, regardless of the consequences for public health. Taking the government's doomed mass testing programme, Operation Moonshot, as its object of analysis, this chapter explores how the desire to save face for unwanted superlatives (e.g., 'the highest death rates in Europe') resulted in a bizarre kind of auto-one-upmanship, with increasingly unrealistic future testing targets set at the same time as previous – and comparatively more modest – targets went unmet. Unlike the original Moonshot, John F. Kennedy's race to put a man on the moon, Operation Moonshot relied on meeting targets which were technically quantifiable but which, to many people, represented an abstract distinction between two large numbers. Like the original Moonshot, however, it tapped into – and fuelled – narratives of national exceptionalism, going in search of a new, flattering superlative, a 'world-beating' test and trace system to allow the UK to posture on the international stage, and retroactively cast Brexit in a more positive light.

Covid-19 and Shame

The reader can be forgiven for thinking that the scenes of shame which accompanied Covid-19 were themselves inevitable. Far from instilling such hopelessness, we intend this book to act as a call for change, for political discourses and public health work which take shame seriously and set out to avoid and reduce it. As Tamson Pietsch and Frances Flanagan argue in their 2020 essay, 'Here We Stand: Temporal Thinking in Urgent Times', much of the capacity of the humanities to disrupt and unsettle lies in our ability to unpick and contextualize phenomena which could otherwise be mistaken as unavoidable or, worse, as 'natural'. Through a shame lens on the pandemic and a humanities lens on shame, the harms we explore 'appear powerful, but also re-makeable'.[61] Taking stock of the UK's public health response to Covid-19 during 2020, therefore, is not just an exercise in recollection and dissection. While these processes are undeniably important, we carry them out to imagine – and articulate – an alternative. This book ends on a note of hope. Shame-sensitive practice is possible in public health, but it has to be a collective endeavour.

Notes

1. Aberforthsgoat, 'To Think I Shouldn't be Named and Shamed for Not Clapping', Mumsnet, 10:17 pm, 22 April 2020. https://www.mumsnet.com/Talk/am_i_being_unreasonable/3888389-To-think-I-shouldnt-be-named-and-shamed-for-not-clapping.

2. Aberforthsgoat, 'To Think'.

3. Lucy Middleton, 'Exhausted Mum "named and shamed" for Sleeping through Clap for Carers', *Metro*, 26 April 2020. https://metro.co.uk/2020/04/26/exhausted-mum-named-shamed-sleeping-clap-carers-12611114/.

4. Julian Baggini, 'The Moralising Spy Next Door – Are You Being Judged?', *Financial Times*, 30 April 2021. https://www.ft.com/content/325d9378-2ac0-4776-9264-ff83bcfa5ef9.

5. Natasha Hinde, 'Final "Clap For Carers" Will Be Tonight, Says Founder. Here's Why', *Huffington Post*, 28 May 2020. https://www.huffingtonpost.co.uk/entry/final-clap-for-carers-will-be-tonight-says-founder-heres-why_uk_5ecf7d32c5b6cbc993fb879b.

6. D. T. Max, 'The Public-Shaming Pandemic', *The New Yorker*, 21 September 2020. https://www.newyorker.com/magazine/2020/09/28/the-public-shaming-pandemic?utm_source=NYR_REG_GATE.

7. Felicity Callard and Elisa Perego, 'How and Why Patients made Long Covid', *Social Science & Medicine* vol. 268 (2021), 113426. 10.1016/j.socscimed.2020.113426.

8. Office for National Statistics, *Deaths involving COVID-19, England and Wales: Deaths Occurring in March 2020*. https://www.ons.gov.uk/peoplepopulationandcommunity/birthsdeathsandmarriages/deaths/bulletins/deathsinvolvingcovid19englandandwales/deathsoccurringinmarch2020.

9. Tedros Adhanon Ghebreyesus, 'WHO Director-General's Opening Remarks at the Media Briefing on COVID-19', *World Health Organization*, 11 March 2020. https://www.who.int/director-general/speeches/detail/who-director-general-s-opening-remarks-at-the-media-briefing-on-covid-19—11-march-2020.

10. Benjamin Mueller and Isabella Kwai, 'For U.K., an Early Taste of Brexit as Borders Are Sealed', *The New York Times*, 21 December 2020. https://www.nytimes.com/2020/12/21/world/europe/brexit-covid-uk.html.

11. UK Health Security Agency, *COVID-19 Confirmed Deaths in England (to 31 December 2020)*, 21 February 2022. https://www.gov.uk/government/publications/covid-19-reported-sars-cov-2-deaths-in-england/covid-19-confirmed-deaths-in-england-to-31-december-2020-report.

12. Des Fitzgerald, 'Stay the Fuck at Home', *Somatosphere*, 13 April 2020. http://somatosphere.net/2020/stay-the-fuck-at-home.html/; Alison Blunt, 'Introduction to Stay Home Stories', 19 February 2021. https://www.stayhomestories.co.uk/introduction-to-stay-home-stories.

13. Ru Jia et al., 'Mental Health in the UK during the COVID-19 Pandemic: Cross-Sectional Analyses from a Community Cohort Study', *BMJ Open,* 2020. 10:e040620. https://doi.org/10.1136/bmjopen-2020-040620.

14. Amelia Tait, 'Pandemic Shaming: Is It Helping Us to Keep Our Distance?', *The Guardian*, 4 April 2020. https://www.theguardian.com/science/2020/apr/04/pandemic-shaming-is-it-helping-us-keep-our-distance; Julia Marcus, 'Quarantine Fatigue Is Real', *The Atlantic*, 11 May 2020. https://www.theatlantic.com/ideas/archive/2020/05/quarantine-fatigue-real-and-shaming-people-wont-help/611482/.

15. Charles Rosenberg, 'What Is an Epidemic? AIDS in Historical Perspective', *Daedalus* vol. 118:2 (1989), 1–17, 7.

16. Rosenberg, 'What is an epidemic?', 7.

17. Martin D. Moore, 'Historicising "Containment and Delay": COVID-19, the NHS and High-risk Patients' [version 1; peer review: 2 approved], *Wellcome Open Research* vol. 5:130 (2020). https://doi.org/10.12688/wellcomeopenres.15962.1.

18. See, for instance, *Thinking in a Pandemic* (Boston: Boston Review, 2020) https://bostonreview.net/special_project/thinking-pandemic-project-page/ and Mary E. Fissell et al., 'Special Issue: Reimaging Epidemics', *Bulletin of the History of Medicine* vol. 94:4 (2020).

19. Thomas J. Scheff, 'Elias, Freud and Goffman: Shame as the Master Emotion', in *The Sociology of Norbert Elias*, eds. Steven Loyal and Stephen Quilley (Cambridge: Cambridge University Press, 2004).

20. Frank Broucek, 'Shame and Its Relationship to Early Narcissistic Developments', *International Journal of Psychoanalysis* vol. 65 (1982), 369.

21. For example, Luna Dolezal, *The Body and Shame: Phenomenology, Feminism and the Socially Shaped Body* (Lanham, MD: Lexington Books, 2015); Dan Zahavi. *Self and Other: Exploring Subjectivity, Empathy and Shame* (Oxford: Oxford University Press, 2014); Helen Lynd. *On Shame and the Search for Identity* (New York: Harcourt Brace, 1958); Michael Lewis, *Shame: The Exposed Self* (New York: The Free Press, 1992).

22. Erving Goffman, *The Presentation of Self in Everyday Life* (Middlesex: Penguin Books, 1959).

23. John Bradshaw, *Healing the Shame That Binds You*. Deerfield Beach (Florida: Health Communications, Inc., 2005). See also: Christine Sanderson, *Counselling Skills for Working with Shame* (London and Philadelphia: Jessica Kingsley Publishers, 2015).

24. For example see: Sanderson, *Counselling Skills for Working with Shame*; Bradshaw, *Healing the Shame that Binds you*; Stephen Pattison, *Shame: Theory, Therapy, Theology* (Cambridge: Cambridge University Press, 2000); Melissa Harris-Perry, *Sister Citizen: Shame, Stereotypes and Black Women in America* (New Haven and London: Yale University Press, 2011); Donald Nathanson, *Shame and Pride: Affect, Sex and the Birth of the Self* (New York: W. W. Norton & Company, 1992); Patricia A. DeYoung, *Understanding and Treating Chronic Shame: A Relational/Neurobiological Approach* (London: Routledge, 2015).

25. Clara Fischer, 'Gender and the Politics of Shame: A Twenty-First-Century Feminist Shame Theory', *Hypatia: A Journal of Feminist Philosophy* vol. 33:3 (2018), 372–83.

26. Sandra Lee Bartky, *Femininity and Domination: Studies in the Phenomenology of Oppression* (London: Routledge, 1990), 96.

27. Uri Friedman, 'Face Masks Are in', *The Atlantic*, 2 April 2020. https://www.theatlantic.com/politics/archive/2020/04/america-asia-face-mask-coronavirus/609283/.

28. Susan S. Williams, '"A Strange, Contagious Fear": Scarlet Letters and Shame in the Time of Coronavirus', *Nathaniel Hawthorne Review* vol. 47:1 (2021), 144–66, 149.

29. W. E. Douglas Creed, Bryant Ashley Hudson, Gerardo A. Okhuysen and Kristin Smith-Crowe, 'Swimming in a Sea of Shame: Incorporating Emotion into Explanations of Institutional Reproduction and Change', *Academy of Management Review* vol. 39:3 (2014), 275–301.

30. Karen Adkins, 'When Shaming Is Shameful: Double Standards in Online Shame Backlashes', *Hypatia* vol. 34:1 (2019), 76–97.

31. 'Let's Stop Clapping for the NHS, Says Woman Who Started the Ritual', *The Guardian*, 16: 25 BST, 22 May 2020. https://www.theguardian.com/world/2020/may/22/lets-stop-clapping-for-the-nhs-says-woman-who-started-the-ritual.

32. Bruce G. Link and Jo C. Phelan, 'Conceptualizing Stigma', *Annual Review of Sociology* 27 (2001), 377.

33. Luna Dolezal, 'Shame, Stigma and HIV: Considering Affective Climates and the Phenomenology of Shame Anxiety', *Lambda Nordica* vols. 2–3 (2021), 48.

34. Graham Scambler, 'Re-Framing Stigma: Felt and Enacted Stigma and Challenges to the Sociology of Chronic and Disabling Conditions.' *Social Theory & Health* vol. 2:1 (2004), 33.

35. Scambler, 'Re-framing Stigma', 33.

36. Scambler, Graham, 'Heaping Blame on Shame: "Weaponizing Stigma" for Neoliberal Times', *The Sociological Review Monographs* vol. 66:4 (2018), 53.

37. For example: Robert Walker, *The Shame of Poverty* (Oxford: Oxford University Press, 2014); Imogen Tyler, *Stigma: The Machinery of Inequality* (London: Zed Books Ltd., 2020).

38. Dolezal, 'Shame, Stigma and HIV', 49.

39. Jane Hand, '"Look after yourself": Visualising Obesity as a Public Health Concern in 1970s and 1980s Britain', in *Balancing the Self: Medicine, Politics and the Regulation of Health in the Twentieth Century*, eds. Mark Jackson and Martin D. Moore (Manchester: Manchester University Press, 2020), 97.

40. Diana Duong, 'Does Shaming Have a Place in Public Health?', *CMAJ: Canadian Medical Association journal = journal de l'Association medicale canadienne* vol. 193:2 (2021), E59–E60. https://doi.org/10.1503/cmaj.1095910.

41. Walker, *The Shame of Poverty*, 52.

42. Alexandra Brewis and Amber Wutich, 'Why We Should Never Do It: Stigma as a Behaviour Change Tool in Global Health', *BMJ Global Health* vol. 4 e001911 (2019). https://doi.org/10.1136/bmjgh-2019-001911.

43. Alexandra Brewis and Amber Wutich, *Lazy, Crazy and Disgusting: Stigma and the Undoing of Global Health* (Baltimore: Johns Hopkins University Press, 2019), 188.

44. Graham Scambler, *A Sociology of Shame and Blame: Insiders versus Outsiders* (Basingstoke: Palgrave Macmillan, 2020), 79.

45. Rowena Mason, 'Boris Johnson Boasted of Shaking Hands on the Day Sage Warned Not to', *The Guardian* 14:22 BST, 5 May 2020, https://www.theguardian.com/politics/2020/may/05/boris-johnson-boasted-of-shaking-hands-on-day-sage-warned-not-to.

46. Roy M Anderson et al., 'COVID-19 Spread in the UK: The End of the Beginning?', *Lancet* vol. 396:10251 (2020), 587–90. https://doi.org/10.1016/S0140-6736(20)31689-5.

47. Scambler, *A Sociology of Shame and Blame*, 2.

48. Scambler, *A Sociology of Shame and Blame*, 79.

49. Roy Coleman and Beka Mullin-McCandlish, 'The Harms of State, Free-Market Common Sense and COVID-19', *State Crime Journal* vol. 10:1 (2021), 170–88. https://doi.org/10.13169/statecrime.10.1.0170.

50. Tyler, *Stigma*, 18.

51. Tyler, *Stigma*, 9.

52. Tyler, *Stigma*, 196–7.

53. Alexandra Homolar and Georg Löfflmann, 'Populism and the Affective Politics of Humiliation Narratives', *Global Studies Quarterly* vol. 1:1 (2021), 1–11. https://doi.org/10.1093/isagsq/ksab002, 2.

54. Homolar and Löfflmann, 'Populism', 2.

55. Tyler, *Stigma*.

56. Rosário Couto Costa, 'The Place of the Humanities in Today's Knowledge Society', *Palgrave Communications* vol. 5:38 (2019). https://doi.org/10.1057/s41599-019-0245-6.

57. Stephen Hinchliffe et al., 'Healthy Publics: Enabling Cultures and Environments for Health', *Palgrave Communications* vol. 4:57 (2018). https://doi.org/10.1057/s41599-018-0113-9.

58. Mass Observation, 'History of Mass Observation', 2015. http://www.massobs.org.uk/about/history-of-mo.

59. Sarah Crowe, Kathrin Cresswell, Ann Robertson, Guro Huby, Anthony Avery and Aziz Sheikh, 'The Case Study Approach'. *BMC Medical Research Methodology* vol. 11 (2011). https://doi.org/10.1186/1471-2288-11-100.

60. On the idea of using a 'shame lens', see Luna Dolezal and Matthew Gibson, 'Beyond a Trauma-Informed Approach and towards Shame-Sensitive Practice', *Humanities and Social Sciences Communications* vol. 9:214 (2022), 1–10.

61. Tamson Pietsch and Frances Flanagan, 'Here We Stand: Temporal Thinking in Urgent Times', *History Australia* vol. 17:2 (2020), 252–71, 260.

CHAPTER 1
COVIDIOTS!: THE LANGUAGE OF PANDEMIC SHAMING

22 March 2020. An image of East London's Columbia Road Flower Market begins to circulate.[1] People are brushing shoulders. To one side, a man, unmasked, sports a tote bag prominently displaying the phrase, 'Too Many Humans'. The BBC's caption is impressively understated: 'shoppers did not always follow the 2m advice'. The same day, a BBC journalist tweets a further image of the crowded market with the somewhat less dry injunction 'STOP THIS NOW'.[2] Later that evening, Boris Johnson formally insists that people 'have to stay two metres apart; you have to follow the social distancing advice'.[3] Although some version of the guidance has been recommended since at least 4 March by Public Health England, this is the first time that Johnson raises it in his own coronavirus statements.[4] Still, the comments on the photos – almost 7000 for the article and 881 for the tweet – are less sedate: 'They can put the flowers on their parents' and grandparents graves, and maybe send some to the families of the health workers they kill'; 'These people are basically biological terrorists. It's criminally insane'; 'People are being so stupid. They are being so selfish.' The overall sentiment is pithily summed up in one short response to the tweeted photo: 'You're kidding?! Covidiots …'[5]

In the backlash that followed the photos' publication, the Columbia Road market organizers were lambasted for what one social media user called their 'really irresponsible behaviour'.[6] Even the health secretary Matt Hancock would describe those who visited crowded places as 'very selfish'.[7] However, the decision to keep the market open was made by the local council. The people visiting the market had not broken any laws or rules. In fact, lockdown rules, including the directive to 'Stay at Home', only came into force the following day. Social distancing guidelines, including the two-metre rule, were still merely guidance, not law. The government's official advice was 'Keep your distance if you go out – 2 metres apart *where possible*'.[8] On the 22nd of March 2020, the government's own advice was that if you were healthy and weren't one of the 1.5 million vulnerable people who required shielding, then you should go outside for exercise. As one market organizer simply put it, 'that's what people were doing'.[9] Nonetheless, the Columbia Road Flower Market became a site of notoriety in international news. On 23 March, an article appeared in Canada's *The National Post* featured the now infamous tweeted photo of the market. It was titled: '#COVIDIOTS gather in large groups despite public health warnings to keep social distance'.[10]

The Columbia Road Flower Market illustrates the ease with which online users turned to shame and blame in response to suspected infractions. Commentators, usually on social media, weighed in with claims impugning the market goers' mental capacity, generosity and public regard. These ritualistic attacks served two functions: they projected the full weight of the pandemic's negative affect on the heads of a few scapegoats, while also positioning the commentators as defenders of the social order. Despite, or, we would argue, because of, the vagaries of public messaging in the early pandemic, people resorted to shame to ensure social cohesion. This seems to be the basic principle behind 'pandemic shaming', the term we used in our Introduction to describe publicly naming, blaming and shaming individuals and groups for not following public health rules, or practicing behaviour seemingly at odds with the needs of the collective (such as hoarding toilet paper or improper hand washing). Then, our aim was simply to introduce incidents of pandemic shaming as surface manifestations of broader patterns of social and political ideologies, policies and power relations.

In this chapter, we focus on the language of pandemic shaming. We pay particular attention to its use of a language of capacity to identify and censure perceived deviations from social norms, and so control and influence individual and collective behaviour. To emphasize the role that language played in this social policing, we turn to a term whose popularity the Columbia Flower Market story helped grow: covidiot. The case of 'covidiot' presents us with an exemplary case of a term whose linguistic 'success' was predicated on a perceived need to name, blame and shame certain behaviour during the pandemic.

The new language of the pandemic

In 2020, 'covidiot' presented one of the pithier forms of naming and shaming. But the first published uses of this neologism were scarcely so prominent. On 26 February, a Twitter user responded to the question 'In the Great Virus Off of 2020, which one are you more worried about?' with a single word: 'COVIDIOT-45'.[11] Another user transformed the term into a hashtag on 1 March 2020: 'trump's new name should be #COVIDIOT and his followers that don't believe in science should be #COVIDIOTS #trumpvirus #COVID19 #CoronaVirus #Science'.[12] Neither of these tweets went viral. The first tweet received twelve likes; the second was retweeted twice. Still, they, like many of other early uses of the term, shared a target and a cause: the forty-fifth president of the United States, Donald J. Trump, for his handling of the Covid-19 pandemic. When the term began to trend on social media in early March, there seemed to be only one covidiot for Anglophone Twitter, and that was Trump. This gave the earliest iterations of the term a political valency: it offered an insult that the otherwise powerless might use as a means to humiliate a powerful individual.

By the time of the Columbia Road market incident, #covidiot had changed. It referred more generally to 'a person who ignores public health advice, thereby putting others at risk'.[13] On 16 March 2020, Urban Dictionary, an online repository of slang, registered the following definition: 'Someone who ignores the warnings regarding public health or safety'.[14] From its initial appearance as a form of fearless speech, calling the powerful to account, the word had morphed into an indictment of pandemic rule breaking by the general public. From March 2020, invoking the neologism 'covidiot', especially on social media, became associated with bids to police behaviour through naming, blaming and shaming.

Terminology is value-laden, particularly in medical, public health and scientific contexts.[15] The words we choose or adopt directly influence how we conceive of phenomena such as diseases, technologies, public health measures and medical interventions.[16] Language provides the logics, metaphors and sense-making through which we understand events, experiences or objects which might be unfamiliar.[17] This has direct consequences for shaping our ethical intuitions, along with behaviour, practice and policy.[18] The new language of the pandemic provided a direct means for influencing and managing our social, emotional and psychological responses to Covid-19. Metaphors (like 'wartime'), epidemiological terminology (such as 'herd immunity', 'contact tracing' and 'R-value') and neologisms ('covidiot') created a shared vocabulary through which we made sense of our new reality.[19] While many of these linguistic developments helped build familiarity, language also legitimated divisive, discriminatory, blaming and shaming practices.[20] Terms such as 'superspreader' or 'patient zero' provided immediate human targets for blame and shame. The widespread use of the terms 'China virus' and 'Wuhan virus' produced racist stigma, while insulating Western countries from blame for spreading of the virus. Neologisms, such as 'covidiot', provided a succinct and memorable means to target and punish individuals.

A comparable slur, 'Typhoid Mary', has its origins in the real-time shaming of Mary Mallon in New York in the early twentieth century. Coined by her fellow domestic staff, 'Typhoid Mary' came via extensive contemporary media coverage to connote anyone ignorantly spreading illness or disease.[21] The epithet performs similar work to 'covidiot', in the sense that it attempts simultaneously to shame and to effect a change in behaviour. As an asymptomatic carrier of Typhoid, Mallon became a byword both for her infectiousness and for her stubborn refusal to conform to medical guidance, as she returned to work – and continued to transmit Typhoid – under an assumed name after a lawyer secured her release from enforced hospital custodianship.[22] Although she would almost certainly have been branded a 'typhoidiot' in 2020, no medical professional seems to have taken the time to adequately convey the complex idea that she could both feel healthy and transmit disease, instead subjecting her to dehumanizing, shaming and carceral interventions, including threatening to remove her gallbladder.[23] As the doctor who first connected her to instances of Typhoid across several homes described his opening conversational gambit: 'I was as diplomatic as possible, but I had to say I suspected her of making people sick and that I wanted specimens of her urine, feces and blood.'[24]

But the emergence of 'covidiot' also fits into a much larger narrative about the development of a novel language to describe the social impacts of the novel coronavirus. In recent years, the analysis of Twitter discourse has become a popular means for following, in real time, public concerns about large scale events.[25] In the case of Covid-19, it has served as a public testing ground for neologisms, or new words, coined to describe circumstances related to the pandemic.[26] In giving names to new realities, notes Amanda Roig-Marín, 'coroneologisms' have helped us to process and endure 'these unprecedented times', and 'highlight the profound interrelation between language and society'.[27] Disease neologisms, of course, are not new; they have emerged, for example, in speech around HIV and AIDS in Botswana in the early 2000s.[28] During Covid-19, terms such as 'quarantini', 'morona', 'maskhole', 'spendemic', and 'ronavation' have developed to provide light relief to the often devastating and highly disruptive realities of the pandemic and lockdowns.[29] Still, these terms hardly emerge from nowhere: 'all of these new lexical terms play with existing words, their sounds and resonance'.[30]

They provide an intuitively accessible repository of terms (a lexicon) that enables rapid, highly specific communication about the pandemic.[31]

In this regard, they parallel the ways conceptual metaphors helped to make sense of the virus. As Elena Semino has argued, the metaphors that arose to describe Covid-19, an unprecedented and complex situation, found their sources in 'an enemy, a mugger, a tsunami, a fire, a race, and even glitter that gets everywhere', images made familiar through media and political discourses.[32] By using intuitively accessible concepts, like journeys, battles or fires, metaphors help to illustrate or explain hitherto unknown conditions. What metaphors do for our understanding, a specific lexicon does for our interpersonal communications. Neologisms, like 'covidiot', formulate new terms out of existing words (in this case, covid + idiot), enabling us to talk to each other with heightened specificity, as fellow initiates into a collective experience. In effect, these neologisms create a new speech community, one whose social understanding is reflected in the facility with which it uses the new language.

Within the context of this emerging language, not all neologisms are treated equally. 'Covidiot' is a singular neologism that demonstrates how, in the new speech community constituted through the pandemic, shaming language enjoyed particular prominence. In the TRAC:COVID dataset, a sampling of more than 84 million tweets composed in English from UK-based accounts between 1 January 2020 and 30 April 2021, #covidiots appears fifth on a list of most frequent hashtags, after #lockdown, #NHS, #staysafe and #pandemic.[33] In other words, covidiot was the most frequently hashtagged coroneologism on Twitter in the UK. This relative prominence can be explained by the term's intuitive clipping and blending of covid and idiot, its easy take up as a hashtag on Twitter and other social media, and the tendency for such hashtags to amplify, as and when they go viral.[34]

It also served a particular function: to enforce or police social behaviours related to lockdown, social distancing and mask wearing.[35] Its six most frequent collocations, or words appearing within the same tweet, were 'people', 'like', 'get', 'one', 'lockdown' and 'mask'. The emphasis on people, lockdown and mask suggests a frequency of declarations about what 'people' should be doing. If this correlation between opinionated declarations and covidiot accusations is true, it certainly conforms to Wicke and Bolognesi's observation that, between March and July 2020, Twitter discourse about the pandemic shifted in emphasis from fact-based to opinion-based messaging.[36] More persuasively, the hashtag most likely to appear with #covidiots was #lockdown, indicating a correlation between being called the former and breaking the rules of the latter. The hashtags most commonly associated with the variation, #covididiots, are even more demonstrative of its use as an injunction: #stayathomesavelives, #coronaviruslockdown and #lockdown. By contrast, the second and third most popular hashtags to appear with #covidiots demonstrate how, even as the term started to be used to shame the general public, it never entirely lost its political force: they were #borisjohnson (the British prime minister) and #toriesout (the ruling political party). These corpus-based responses give a sense of how #covidiots was being mobilized as a tool of pandemic shaming, in a discursive period that was marked by interpersonal, opinion-based invective.

However, the term 'covidiot' didn't just circulate on social media as an informal means of censuring individuals. The term became favoured by journalists and the media as a shorthand to report pandemic shaming or to engage in it. A spate of news stories used 'covidiot' to describe people associated with actions that, under the exceptional circumstances of the pandemic and lockdown, were seen as social threats and acts of gross irresponsibility. Relatively early in the history of its usage, the local media outlets that furnished readers with a steady diet of covidiot stories began to drop their inverted commas, presenting the term in a matter-of-fact, straightforward way.[37] The perpetrators of minor public health transgressions weren't 'covidiots', they were covidiots; their culpability and the term itself were no longer provisional or up for debate.

In headlines and copy, attempts were made to draw out potentially humorous aspects of the subject's behaviour. A representative example was the Somerset County Gazette's 'Covidiots drove to Dartmoor because 'they don't like Taunton".[38] Focusing on the explanation that the 'covidiots' gave to police, the article plays on the shared assumption that not liking Taunton is not an excuse for driving to Dartmoor. In addition to breaking lockdown rules, they were comically incapable of convincing the police. As with so many of these 'covidiot' pieces, a bland formulation of right and wrong papers over serious questions of access, power and pandemic citizenship. For people under lockdown in urban environments, even pleasant county towns, nearby areas of natural beauty, with fresh air, few people and wide open spaces, undoubtedly exerted a considerable pull. 'Don't like' reads as petulant, but it may have articulated a genuine and pressing psychological need. In a journalistic mill where the identification of 'covidiots' very often resulted directly from police action, this form of media shaming is inextricable from deeper problems of social capital, racism, heteronormativity and class.

If you are (the kind of person who is) able to convince a member of the police that your behaviour is legitimate or an honest mistake, then you are not a 'covidiot' but a 'good citizen'.[39]

Calling someone a covidiot

What does it mean to call someone an idiot in public? Whether directed at Donald J. Trump, a neighbour stockpiling toilet paper or a Dartmoor walker, the act of calling someone an idiot has a specific function: it identifies the person as someone with questionable mental capacity or diminished common sense. The aim is to indict them for something they are doing, have done or have failed to do, and so persuade them to feel something about their act or omission and/or prompt them to change their behaviour. Importantly, 'idiots' function as 'a category of people against whom we rational modern (and post-modern) folk can identify ourselves, to affirm our intelligence and to assert our claims to respect and justice'.[40] Although idiot was understood to be 'ignorant' and 'uneducated' in Greek and Latin, the word developed a specific, technical meaning in eugenic, psychiatric and legal theories of capacity in the late nineteenth and early twentieth centuries.[41] These 'modern' uses of 'idiot' carry particularly offensive connotations related to intellectual disability. And yet, despite sharing a similar history with other terms which are now fully discredited, 'idiot' has never quite received the same ethical censure, in part because it is often folded into celebrated figures like the holy fool.[42]

Still, most of us would prefer not to be called idiots. Certainly, we don't like to have our mental capacity challenged, or to be seen or labelled by others as mentally deficient or incompetent. Being designated 'an idiot' is stigmatizing; it undermines our standing within society as well as inducing shame, or a negative self-conscious emotional experience as a result of having failed to live up to the standards of others, one's community or one's broader society.[43] Because being called an idiot is shaming, we generally go to great lengths, both consciously and unconsciously, to avoid actions and behaviour that may plausibly elicit accusations of idiocy. We don't want to be called an idiot, because we don't want to experience shame and stigma, and all the related social phenomena, such as discrimination, status-loss and marginalization, that usually come hand-in-hand with being marked out as inferior, deficient, unworthy or damaged.

If calling someone an idiot communicates a failure to live up to the standards of the community, with the intention of shaming them, what does the blending of idiot with 'covid' do? Quite simply, it ties these standards to the singular conditions of the pandemic. Accordingly, it serves to shame behaviour that violates the extraordinary standards of behaviour and practice that communities and societies developed in response to the crisis. If I call someone a 'covidiot', this designation first of all serves to call out someone's bad behaviour, and at the same time also serves to mark myself as not a covidiot. Shaming and blaming others is an attempt to insulate the self from shame and blame, while at the same time serving to alleviate diffuse feelings of anxiety and fear by pinning them directly onto an individual.[44]

These dynamics are neatly illustrated by paralleling the UK government's announcements with spikes or surges in the incidence of #covidiot or #covididiot in tweets by UK-based Twitter users. In the TRAC:COVID dataset, the terms surged when the government announced the first and second lockdowns and, as importantly, the easing of measures. As norms over socially acceptable behaviour changed, and new boundaries for what was appropriate or not were demarcated, there was a concomitant flurry of activity to emphasize the ways these boundaries would be socially policed. Interestingly, the single biggest spike occurred on the day that the government changed its public health message, from 'Stay at Home, Protect the NHS, Save Lives' to 'Stay Alert, Protect the NHS, Save Lives', on 10 May 2020.

To understand why, we need to recall the role that 'Stay Home, Protect the NHS, Save Lives' played as the official public health message during the UK's first national lockdown. First alluded to in the prime minister's statement on coronavirus of the 23rd of March, it followed weeks of non-committal and often murky and confusing 'advice', 'recommendation' and 'suggestion' that people should follow social distancing guidance.[45] By contrast, the Stay Home campaign emphasized, with striking clarity, what needed to be done ('Stay at Home') to achieve certain desired outcomes ('Protect the NHS, Save Lives'). Using a bright red-and-yellow colour scheme (a colour combination that routinely conveys warnings, emergencies, hazards or prohibitions), full-page advertisements were placed in most national newspapers and a social media campaign was launched. The campaign featured images of NHS staff in face masks and other personal protective equipment, looking directly out at the viewer. Blame and shame were conveyed implicitly in the healthcare worker's unflinching and accusatory gaze directed to the viewer, and more explicitly in the slogan accompanying the image: 'If you go out, you can spread it, people will die.' The implication, of course, is that the individual viewing the ad is potentially to blame for spreading the virus and should feel shame for potentially causing illness or death, further burdening overworked NHS workers. Certainly, the emphasis on individual responsibility empowered some to identify others as covidiots for failing to abide by what seemed to be clear injunctions.[46] So why, then, did a softening of the rules lead to a spike in covidiot usage?

The change from 'Stay at Home' to 'Stay Alert' substituted a concrete command enforceable by law with a more abstract imperative. Abstractions rely on personal judgement or common sense about acceptable standards of behaviour. These standards were in a state of flux: the change in messaging accompanied an easing of restrictions. But, if anything, public consensus seemed to suggest a general unwillingness to exit the conditions of lockdown too quickly. Coming soon after pictures of people celebrating VE Day went viral, the invitation to use personal judgement ('Stay Alert') over definite action ('Stay at Home') seemed to demand a supplementary campaign to police that judgement. There were many cases of individuals behaving in reckless and inappropriate ways during the pandemic, flouting and breaking rules such that they created public health risks for others. Other cases can be better explained by this considerable muddiness about what was mandatory and what was recommended or voluntary. Vague injunctions such as 'Stay Alert' meant a lack of clarity about which behaviours were appropriate or expected.

Such cases gesture to the way that articulated and implicit standards of behaviour fit into a larger ecology of language, or interactions between language and its environment.[47] Government announcements played an important role in influencing standards, but their importance was heightened or dampened by other actors in the language environment. In the early days of the pandemic, the government found itself under pressure to underwrite forms of behaviour that large swathes of the UK population had already decided to follow, such as social distancing and mask wearing. Reluctant to commit to an official national lockdown, the government found itself forced into the measure by the accumulated force of social, cultural and economic leaders, their organizations and the general public. As the change from 'Stay at Home' to 'Stay Alert' suggests, community censure through acts of pandemic shaming appeared most strongly at moments when the government's standards allowed for greater ambiguity in interpretation with regard to rules and guidance. Critically, the injunctions not to be a covidiot show how the community sought to police these standards themselves, when government policies were ambiguous and open to interpretation. In Chapter 5, we elaborate on the injunction to apply 'good solid British common sense' to personal behaviour, which, in lieu of clear government guidelines, made unnecessary room for shame and shaming. 'Covidiot' emerged as its complement: a tool for shaming those that didn't show enough common sense. This was exacerbated by the vastly expanded scope for public censure offered by social media; its reliance on the real-time interactions of its users and the simultaneous and virtually instantaneous communication of events to all parts of the world meant that this form of censure could consolidate itself as the generalized term of opprobrium in the Anglophone world.

Stigma and pandemic language

In tandem with broader social and political landscapes, pandemics have historically inflamed logics of 'us versus them', where attempts to deflect and shift blame for contagion and infection have led to the use of shaming language practices. During 2020, populist leaders cultivated shaming language through associating nations, particularly China, with the illness. Terms like 'Wuhan Virus', 'China Virus' and 'Kung Flu' implicitly blamed China for the origin of the virus, while the later emergence of 'Plague Island' served to describe the UK's poor handling of the epidemic.[48] As new variants emerged, they were identified with countries or counties of origin: the South African, Brazilian, UK (or Kent) and Indian variants. The decision to change these designations to letters from the Greek alphabet stemmed in no small way from a desire to deflect stigma, taking valuable lessons from the experiences of people with Asian heritage in the early days of the pandemic.

This, too, appears to fit in a longer history of labelling epidemics by their purported point of origin: the so-called Spanish Flu of 1918 being a striking example. Certainly, we know now that contemporary perceptions about the origins of the 1918 Influenza stemmed in no small way from Spain's neutrality during the First World War: less concerned with the impact of the Influenza on morale, Spanish newspapers were more open about the rise in cases in the early pandemic.[49] Unsurprisingly, the 1918 Influenza was given a different nickname in Spain: it was known as the Naples Soldier, after a 1916 operetta.[50] Its heteronymity continued: in Senegal it was the Brazilian Flu, while in Brazil it was the German Flu. And yet, the apparent continuities belie a striking difference. Importantly, the identification of the Influenza with Spain does not seem to have resulted in any overt stigmatization of Spanish citizens. If anything, German citizens were more likely to be stigmatized.[51] Knowledge about the pandemic's country of origin did not lead, automatically, to the development of stigma when dealing with its citizens, perhaps in part because the orientalist component of shaming in recent respiratory pandemics was absent. These circumstances are all the more compelling when compared with Covid-19, where such stigma was not only allowed to emerge but often repeated and reinforced by persons in positions of power. Although shaming language is more likely to develop during pandemics, it does not have to. So what happened?

The linguistic success of covidiot can be explained by this confluence of circumstances. When it was coined to refer to Donald Trump, it did not simply emerge *ex nihilo*. Rather, it relied upon a historical tendency to portray Trump as morally and intellectually deficient throughout his candidacy for, and eventual elevation to, the US presidency.[52] Seen in this light, the neologism owed its first success to the ease with which it fitted into an existing paradigm, as a novel shorthand for describing an existing situation. That said, and despite frequent efforts to guide or regulate its use, language is determined by the totality of its users. This means that a word coined for one purpose can be, and frequently is, repurposed for other ends. Covidiot lent itself to this repurposing, since its primary function – to shame and censure – resonated with the blame narrative of populism, the personal responsibility narrative of neoliberalism and the impurity narrative of illness, respectively.[53] However politically engaged its initial aims, the term eventually drifted from targeting the powerful to targeting those less powerful. This drift is hardly surprising. In Chapter 3, we show how historically disadvantaged communities, communities whose visibility has often gone hand in hand with political marginality, are more likely to be the recipients of shaming language. With the new resources offered by the term, in conditions where approbation became synonymous with public service, those targeted became those less likely to speak back. Further, those likely to be shamed are also those who have, historically, been shamed in the past, and so are more likely to be shame-prone, or have a justifiable tendency to interpret even ambiguous or ambivalent communication as shaming directed at them.

This raises the stakes for apparently innocent uses of 'covidiot'. And yet, there is a basic dilemma that faces any serious attempt to think about this word, whose attractiveness stems in no small way from its fundamental silliness. Many of its users would defend its use, not merely as generally or socially necessary but as basically humorous, causing little if any actual harm. This explains why, within months of the term becoming popular, at least two self-published collections of anecdotes, detailing the humorous escapades of 'covidiots', could be found on Amazon.[54] These playful narratives present generic stories of 'covidiocy' as benign infractions by actors who survive their adventures unscathed. By contrast, more intimate accounts of the experience show real and persisting feelings of shame in people 'called out' for their behaviour. So, by way of conclusion, we will look at three different stories about covidiots: two focus on politicians who 'avoided' shame and the third looks at ordinary interactions. For all the apparent innocence of the term, its emotional impact is ultimately muted or elevated by the relative distance of the narrators to their respective 'covidiots'.

In *Covidiots: Stories of Idiotic Acts and Bizarre Behaviour* (2020), Steven Harris and Natalia Gómez Álvarez take aim at Boris Johnson's reckless behaviour in the early pandemic, citing his prominent absences from key COBRA meetings in January and February and his boast, on visiting a hospital, that he 'shook hands with everybody'.[55] Written while Johnson was still in intensive care at St Thomas' Hospital, the authors 'sincerely wish him the very best for a full and speedy recovery', while observing how 'little respect' the virus has for 'a go-it-alone attitude and the great British resolve'.[56] In Chapters 5 and 6, we address this attitude in greater detail, especially as it relates to common sense and hyperbolic rhetoric. For the moment, however, we highlight how, by implying Johnson is a 'covidiot', Harris and Gómez Álvarez call into question their 'sincere' best wishes. Belief in someone's sincerity seldom benefits from their making explicit claims to it. By juxtaposing Johnson's past actions with his (then) current medical condition, the authors emphasize that their wishes, sincere or not, are mediated by their sense that he got what he deserved. Moreover, the relative paucity of details ensures that the reader maintains a necessary distance from Johnson, so that he can be dismissed as a covidiot. Harris and Gómez Álvarez are 'shaming up': using their publication to call to account people in positions of power and authority, like Johnson. But, by linking Johnson to more general acts of covidiocy, they are entrenching the term, and the form of shaming it implies, as a socially acceptable form of moral arbitration that establishes a distance from the people it judges.

On the 22 May, newspapers broke the story that Dominic Cummings, the prime minister's senior advisor, had broken lockdown.[57] Subsequent stories clarified successive infractions, first by driving to Durham on 27 March and then in subsequent trips to Barnard Castle (12 April) and to London (13 April).[58] Twitter saw a marked increase in activity juxtaposing references to Cummings and to covidiot.[59] Posts highlighted the difference in standards, a point the Opposition would consolidate in the phrase: 'One rule for them, another for everyone else'. Covidiot, it seemed, had returned, albeit briefly, to its politicized roots. These attempts to shame Cummings worked, insofar as they prompted him to make an unprecedented public explanation. But the lack of apology, or any notable signs of contrition, left many feeling unsatisfied. The overall result was a 'Cummings effect': a loss of confidence in the government and trust in government decision-making.[60] Shame, it seems, had failed to find its mark.

More poignant accounts of shame actually landing are found in the UK's Mass Observation project. When, in the summer of 2020, many British people went to the beach, pictures of scant social distancing led to a massive backlash at peoples' 'covidiocy'. At the same time, however, more shame-prone members of the community reported feeling shame, even though they have not committed any infractions themselves. In an account from Bexhill-on-Sea, a woman considers how this influenced her habitual relationships, even though neither was involved in the incident:

> I went out on Tuesday, with my son, to buy stamps. I sensed a slight hostility. People who would usually smile and let you through a door now avoid eye contact and stay their distance. The woman working in the Post Office was expressing her anger at people who had congregated on the beach the previous day. She hadn't seen it herself, she said; but it was on Facebook (it must be true!) She said they were idiotic. It differed from her usual affable small-talk and it made me un-easy. I said we had been ourselves on Sunday and there was no-one around.[61]

The need to defend herself against potential reflected shame shows how even those without any relation to a particular incident may interpret the act of naming idiots as directed against them. In a moment when shaming has become generally accepted, its potential victims extend beyond those who commit infractions and those who call them out to include anyone who anticipates their own potential implication.

Pandemic shaming was rife in the early pandemic. From April 2020, journalists began to link isolated instances of personal shaming together to address a broader concern with public responses. These often looked to the psychological literature for reasons why shaming behaviour proved so popular. Such reasons ranged from a general sense of *schadenfreude* on the part of the shamers, through their need to regain a sense of control lost through mandatory lockdowns, to the affordances brought about by increased time online. Rather than address this psychological literature, we have chosen to focus on the language that pandemic shaming takes. By tracing the use of covidiot, we have established how the word itself produced certain effects. In no small way, having a word that could function as an easy shorthand for pandemic shaming contributed to further pandemic shaming.

In certain situations, when rules of politeness are suspended, people may be insulted without causing undue shame. In 2001, Sandra Harris observed that traditional rules of politeness were suspended during Prime Minister's Questions, a time allocated by the UK parliament for addressing issues to the current prime minister.[62] This 'systematic impoliteness' was sanctioned, even endorsed, by Members of Parliament because it met dominant expectations of what the speech context demanded. This also meant that moments which might otherwise lead to emotional distress could be understood as coded by the requirements of the situation: shaming language could be used without people feeling shame.

Although the pandemic called rules of politeness into question, speech situations tended to generate the opposite conditions. Even minor infractions were treated as if they would have major implications. This raised the bar for standards of politeness, and, by extension, increased the chances that even quite minor language could be taken as shaming. A term like covidiot, which appears quite silly, ended up having detrimental effects on those it named or even those who felt it might stick to them. This, of course, had its precedents. But, the age of immediate communication meant that this language could be used for multiple shaming events very soon after being coined, and specifically to target infractions related to the pandemic. This generated unprecedented opportunities for shame to be thrown, and to land, often with unintended results. Tracing the use of covidiot through the early pandemic provides a snapshot of the way that pandemic shaming disseminated through the general public. It shows how language adapted to accommodate shaming practices, often by holding those judged at arm's length. While certain behaviours were generally sanctioned, the ease with which the term migrated shows how it demonstrated a proliferation of shame in general, rather than being tied to any particular group or action. But clearly certain groups experienced more shaming than others. In our next two chapters, we look first at the tendency to shame healthcare providers and then at the attachment of particular racial epithets to Covid-19.

Notes

1. 'Coronavirus: Stay at Home to Stay Safe, 1.5 million Advised', *BBC News*, 22 March 2020. https://www.bbc.co.uk/news/uk-51991887.

2. Dino Sofos, 'STOP THIS NOW. Columbia Road Flower Market, East London. Photo Taken Just Now by My Colleague @JJ_Bryant (who was not there as a punter)'. Twitter, 12:06 p.m., 22 March 2020. https://twitter.com/dinosofos/status/1241697657690734593.

3. Boris Johnson, 'Prime Minister's Statement on Coronavirus (COVID-19): 22 March 2020', *Prime Minister's Office, No. 10 Downing Street*. https://www.gov.uk/government/speeches/pm-statement-on-coronavirus-22-march-2020.

4. UK Health Security Agency, 'Coronavirus (COVID-19): What Is Social Distancing?', *UK Health Security Agency Blog*, 4 March 2020. https://ukhsa.blog.gov.uk/2020/03/04/coronavirus-covid-19-what-is-social-distancing/.

5. 'Stay at Home'; Dino Sofos.

6. [Deleted], 'The Columbia Road Flower Market's Twitter Account Has Been Locked Down. Probably Getting a Lot of Backlash about This. Really Irresponsible Behaviour by the Organisers', *Reddit*, 7:45pm, 22 March 2020. https://www.reddit.com/r/london/comments/fmzlr7/columbia_road_flower_market/fl7ozmp/?utm_source=reddit&utm_medium=web2x&context=3.

7. Amelia Tait, 'Pandemic Shaming: Is It Helping Us Keep Our Distance?', *The Guardian*, 4 April 2020. https://amp.theguardian.com/science/2020/apr/04/pandemic-shaming-is-it-helping-us-keep-our-distance.

8. UKHSA, 'Social Distancing'.

9. Tait, 'Pandemic Shaming'.

10. Valerie Dittrich, '#COVIDIOTS Gather in Large Groups despite Public Health Warnings to Keep Social Distance', *The National Post*, 24 March 2020. https://nationalpost.com/news/covidiots-continue-to-gather-in-large-groups-despite-public-health-officials-urging-social-distancing.

11. Rebecca Newell, 'COVIDIOT-45', Twitter, 1:47 p.m., 26 February 2020. https://twitter.com/rebeccanewell7/status/1232663460380631040.

12. Rochelle94965, 'trump's new name should be #COVIDIOT and his followers that don't believe in science should be #COVIDIOTS #trumpvirus #COVID19 #CoronaVirus #Science', Twitter, 12:38 a.m., 1 March 2020. https://twitter.com/Rochelle94965/status/1233914353583177729.

13. Amanda Roig-Marín, 'English-based Coroneologisms', *English Today* vol. 37, 4 (2021), 193.

14. you'reandidiot, 'Covidiot', *Urban Dictionary*, 16 March 2020. https://www.urbandictionary.com/define.php?term=Covidiot.

15. Luna Dolezal, 'The Metaphors of Commercial Surrogacy', in *New Feminist Perspectives on Embodiment*, eds. Luna Dolezal and Clara Fischer (Basingstoke: Palgrave MacMillan, 2018), 221.

16. George Lakoff and Mark Johnson, *Metaphors We Live By* (Chicago: University of Chicago Press, 2003), 214.

17. Lakoff and Johnson, *Metaphors*, 4.

18. Lakoff and Johnson, *Metaphors*, 193.

19. Philipp Wicke and Marianna M. Bolognesi, 'Framing COVID-19: How We Conceptualize and Discuss the Pandemic on Twitter', *PLoS-ONE* vol. 15:9 (2020), e0240010. https://doi.org/10.1371/journal.pone.0240010; Robert Lawson, 'Coronavirus Has Led to an Explosion of New Words and Phrases – and That Helps Us Cope', *The Conversation*, 28 April 2020. https://theconversation.com/coronavirus-has-led-to-an-explosion-of-new-words-and-phrases-and-that-helps-us-cope-136909.

20. On discursive othering during the pandemic, see Martina Berrocal et al., 'Constructing Collective Identities and Solidarity in Premiers' Early Speeches on COVID-19: A Global Perspective', *Humanities and Social Sciences Communications* vol. 8 (2021), 1–12. https://doi.org/10.1057/s41599-021-00805-x.

21. George A. Soper, 'The Curious Career of Typhoid Mary', *Bulletin of the New York Academy of Medicine* vol. 15:10 (1939), 698–712, 710.

22. Filio Marineli et al., 'Mary Mallon (1869–1938) and the History of Typhoid Fever', *Annals of Gastroenterology* vol. 26:2 (2013), 132–4.

23. Janet Brooks, 'The Sad and Tragic Life of Typhoid Mary', *CMAJ: Canadian Medical Association journal = journal de l'Association medicale canadienne* vol. 154:6 (1996), 915–16.

24. Soper, 'The Curious Career of Typhoid Mary', 704.

25. Axel Bruns and Katrin Weller, 'Twitter as a First Draft of the Present: And the Challenges of Preserving It for the Future', *WebSci* vol. 16 (May 2016), 183–9. https://dl.acm.org/doi/10.1145/2908131.2908174.

26. Tatiana Tkacukova, Matt Gee, Andrew Kehoe, Robert Lawson, and Mark McGlashan, *Government Management of the COVID-19 Communication and Public Perception of the Pandemic*. Working Paper (Birmingham: Birmingham City University, 2021).

27. Roig-Marín, 'Coroneologisms', 194.

28. H. M. Batibo and M. M. Kopi, 'A Sociolinguistic Study of the Euphemistic and Idiomatic Expressions Used in HIV/AIDS Speech in Setswana', *Journal of Linguistics and Language in Education* vol. 6 (2004), 1–20.

29. Tonya Byron and Mark Honigsbaum, 'The Language of the Pandemic', *Word of Mouth*, BBC Radio 4, 20 July 2020. https://www.bbc.co.uk/programmes/m000kv7l.

30. Roig-Marín, 'Coroneologisms', 194.

31. Ashraf R. Abdullah and Ameen A. D. Abdulmaged, 'Coronapedia: A Corpus-Driven Analysis of COVID-19 Newspeak and Implications for Language Change', Adab Al-Rafidain Journal, vol. 52:90 (2022), forthcoming.

32. Elena Semino, 'Not Soldiers but Fire-fighters' – Metaphors and Covid-19', *Health Communication* vol. 36:1 (2021), 50–8.

33. Andrew Kehoe, Matt Gee, Robert Lawson, Mark McGlashan, and Tatiana Tkacukova, *TRAC:COVID – Trust and Communication: A Coronavirus Online Visual Dashboard* (2021). Available online at https://traccovid.com.

34. Abdullah and Abdulmaged, 'Coronapedia'. On amplification, see Andrew Peck, 'A Problem of Amplification: Folklore and Fake News in the Age of Social Media', *Journal of American Folklore* vol. 133:529 (2020), 329–51.

35. Tkacukova et al., 'Government Management', 6.

36. Philipp Wicke and Marianna M. Bolognesi, 'Covid-19 Discourse on Twitter: How the Topics, Sentiments, Subjectivity, and Figurative Frames Changed over Time', *Frontiers in Communication* vol. 6 (2021), 651997. doi: 10.3389/fcomm.2021.651997.

37. 'COVIDIOT CAPERS: Latest on Coronavirus Stupidity', *Toronto Sun*, 30 April 2020. https://torontosun.com/news/world/covidiot-capers-latest-on-coronavirus-stupidity. Chris Daniels, 'How brands and agencies are avoiding covidiot influencers', *PR Weekly*, 1 May 2020. https://www.prweek.com/article/1682071/brands-agencies-avoiding-covidiot-influencers.

38. Phil Hill, 'Covidiots Drove to Dartmoor because "they don't like Taunton"', *Somerset County Gazette*, 1 March 2021. https://www.somersetcountygazette.co.uk/news/19125394.covidiots-drove-dartmoor–dont-like-taunton/.

39. Benjamin Weil, 'The "Good" Coronavirus Citizen, the "Covidiot", and the Privilege of #StayAtHome', *Discover Society*, 1 April 2020. https://archive.discoversociety.org/2020/04/01/the-good-coronavirus-citizen-the-covidiot-and-the-privilege-of-stayathome/.

40. Patrick McDonagh, *Idiocy: A Cultural History* (Liverpool: Liverpool University Press, 2015), 2.

41. McDonagh, *Idiocy*, 9; 10.

42. McDonagh, *Idiocy*, 22.

43. Martha Nussbaum, *Hiding from Humanity: Disgust, Shame and the Law* (Princeton: Princeton University Press, 2004), 219.

44. Nussbaum, *Hiding*, 219.

45. 'The Guardian View on the UK's Covid-19 Response: Confused and Hesitant', *The Guardian* (editorial), 15 March 2020, 18.32 GMT. https://www.theguardian.com/commentisfree/2020/mar/15/the-guardian-view-on-the-uks-covid-19-response-confused-and-hesitant.

46. Claude-Hélène Mayer and Elisabeth Vanderheiden, 'Transforming Shame in the Pandemic: An International Study', *Frontiers in Psychology* vol. 12 (2021): 641076, 7.

47. Einar Haugen, *The Ecology of Language* (Stanford: Stanford University Press, 1972), 325.

48. See Chapter 3.

49. Antoni Trilla, Guillem Trilla and Carolyn Daer, 'The 1918 "Spanish Flu" in Spain', *Clinical Infectious Diseases* vol. 47:5 (2008), 668.

50. Trilla, Trilla and Daer, 'The 1918 "Spanish Flu"', 669.

51. Alan M. Kraut, 'Immigration, Ethnicity, and the Pandemic', *Public Health Reports* 125, Supplement 3 (2010), 126.

52. Michael T. Taussig, 'Trump Studies', Hot Spots, *Fieldsights*, 18 January 2017. https://culanth.org/fieldsights/trump-studies.

53. See our Introduction for our discussion of these narratives in relation to pandemic shaming.

54. Steven Harris and Natalia Gómez Álvarez, *Covidiots: Stories of Idiotic Acts and Bizarre Behaviour* (np: Harris and Gómez, 2020); Christina Thé, *Diary of a Former Covidiot* (Singapore: Marshall Cavendish Editions, 2020).

55. Harris and Gómez Álvarez, *Covidiots,* 70.

56. Harris and Gómez Álvarez, *Covidiots,* 71.

57. Matthew Weaver, 'Pressure on Dominic Cummings to Quit over Lockdown Breach', *The Guardian*, 22 March 2020. https://www.theguardian.com/politics/2020/may/22/dominic-cummings-durham-trip-coronavirus-lockdown.

58. Archie Bland, 'Dominic Cummings Timeline', *The Guardian*, 24 May 2020. https://www.theguardian.com/politics/2020/may/24/dominic-cummings-timeline-what-we-know-about-his-movements.

59. Kehoe et al., TRAC: COVID.

60. Daisy Fancourt, Andrew Steptoe and Liam Wright, 'The Cummings Effect: Politics, Trust, and Behaviours during the COVID-19 Pandemic', *The Lancet* vol. 396:10249 (2020), 464–645.

61. Mass Observation Archive (University of Sussex): Replies to 2020 Special Directive [D7105].

62. Sandra Harris, 'Being Politically Impolite, Extending Politeness Theory to Adversarial Political Discourse', *Discourse & Society* vol. 12:4 (2001), 451–72.

CHAPTER 2
SUPER-SPREADERS: SHAMING
HEALTHCARE PROFESSIONALS

7 March 2020. Jenny Mikakos, then health minister for the Australian state of Victoria, declares in a public talk that she is 'flabbergasted that a doctor that has flu-like symptoms has presented to work', treating seventy patients, including two in a care home. The commitment is laudable, she acknowledges, but 'it is irresponsible for people to be going to work if they are unwell'. Later, she opines that his decision to go to work with any symptoms was negligent and should perhaps be referred to the Australian Health Practitioner Regulation Agency, the equivalent to the UK's General Medical Council.[1]

Although Mikakos does not name the doctor, she does mention his surgery and his recent trip to the United States. Journalists are quick to identify a Melbourne-based GP, Chris Higgins, who had recently returned from a trip to the United States with a runny nose. In his own account, Higgins explains why he did not meet the criteria for Covid-19 testing set by Mikakos's own office when he returned to Australia:

> I had a mild cold when I returned from the USA last Saturday morning which had almost resolved itself by Monday morning, hence my decision to return to work. I hesitated to do a swab because I did not fulfil your criteria for testing but did one anyway on Thursday evening… not imagining for one moment it would turn out to be positive.[2]

While Higgins ceased working and notified all his patients after he tested positive, the immediate reputation damage from the media attention that followed compromised his practice and his livelihood.

Mikakos's comments initially provoked pandemic shaming directed at Dr Higgins on social media, with comments on Twitter such as: 'Personally

I'm "flabbergasted" at Dr Chris Higgins arrogance.… Seeing 70 clinic patients and then visiting a Nursing home, shame on him.' But a shame backlash quickly ensued. Mikakos found herself the target of online shaming, particularly from the Australian medical community. Numerous posts were made by prominent Australian medics defending Higgins and shaming Mikakos in turn for undermining confidence in Australia's doctors. More than 11,000 people signed a petition calling for Mikakos to officially apologize, while #IStandWithChrisHiggins and #Flabbergaslighting trended on social media.[3]

Jenny Mikakos's attempt to publicly shame Dr Chris Higgins for being a Covid-19 'super-spreader' was by no means an isolated phenomenon during 2020.[4] In the international media, there were several high-profile cases of healthcare workers being shamed for inadvertently carrying the virus to others, even when there were no proven cases of infection. In Poland, Dr Wojciech Rokita was publicly shamed after travelling to a car dealership while awaiting the results of a Covid test, which turned out to be positive. Named in the comments section of an online tabloid, Rokita was subjected to phone calls, hate mail and personal attacks, even from friends and former patients. On 18 March 2020, he committed suicide, hanging himself in his hospital room.[5] In Canada, Dr Jean-Robert Ngola was shamed online for supposedly violating the New Brunswick Emergency Measures Act, by not initially self-isolating after a routine border crossing from Quebec. Ngola's shaming was inflected with racist vitriol, and the threat of criminal proceedings – later withdrawn – underscored his precarious status as a racialized doctor.[6]

In the UK, even as they were applauded (both literally and metaphorically) for their 'heroic' efforts, healthcare workers were subjected to significant amounts of shaming, fear and stigma. This primarily resulted from widespread PPE shortages and inadequate testing which meant that there were significant risks of contagion associated with the caring professions, particularly those working on the 'frontline' of hospitals and care homes. The vitriol behind the shaming was fuelled by the often superhuman expectations that land on healthcare workers, that they should not only *know* better but *do* better, and also be impervious to the illnesses and frailties that plague ordinary people. The case of Chris Higgins ended 'well', we might say, insofar as there was a shame backlash, and he won over public opinion and had the unwavering support of his professional community. For other doctors and healthcare workers, Covid-19 shaming was personally and professionally harmful, and sometimes even devastating. This chapter explores how the shaming and stigmatization of healthcare professionals became commonplace during 2020, and the various circumstances and forces that coalesced to make this an ordinary phenomenon.

Healthcare worker shaming in past pandemics

The stigma associated with disease is experienced as shame by individuals and groups who are perceived to carry or spread it. In almost all human cultures, there is shame attached to being 'contaminated', to the vulnerability inherent in illness and to potentially spreading a disease to others. While there have been outpourings of support and admiration for healthcare workers 'fighting on the frontline' of Covid-19, their experiences also form part of a long global history of shame and stigma around the medical professionals who respond to disease and tend those who are infected or ill.

In previous epidemics and pandemics, healthcare workers have been shunned, feared and treated with suspicion. Outbreaks of the bubonic plague in the late seventeenth century were accompanied by popular hostility towards both the sinister 'Beak Doctors' in mainland Europe and the 'plague-nurses' providing palliative care to sufferers in London in 1665. The German engraver Paul Fürst depicted young people fleeing a plague doctor in a 1656 print; the accompanying text includes the lines 'He seeks cadavers to eke out a living/Just like the raven on the dung heap'.[7] In London, nurses were implicated in the spread of plague, as contemporaries accused them of 'secretly convey[ing] the pestilent taint from sores of the infected to those who were well'. Stories circulated of their ghoulish opportunism, with one nurse supposedly 'crushed under the weight of goods she had stolen from a plague victim'.[8]

Anxieties over healthcare workers as sources of contagion further mingled with conspiratorial thinking, class struggle and perceptions of profiteering in European cholera riots over the nineteenth and early twentieth centuries.[9] In Britain, riots in Liverpool and Totnes were organized around the belief that cholera victims were being murdered by doctors for use in anatomical dissection, reflecting a broader medical and moral debate over appropriate uses of the dead.[10] Communities in Russia and Italy rejected medical aid and attacked or threatened doctors and nurses, convinced that they were responsible for 'the wilful spread of disease'.[11] In each of these cases, confused narratives over the intentional or unintentional spread of disease were collapsed into anger over motives which seemed ulterior to care, whether professional or financial. Some of these anxieties were mirrored in Covid-19, as medical professionals were shamed both for their physical proximity to the virus and through allegations that they were using the pandemic to advance particular political causes, sow disinformation or seek personal notoriety and attention.

More recently, shame and stigma around healthcare workers has been a recurring feature in social and relational responses to viruses such as HIV, SARS and Ebola. One doctor working on HIV wards in Britain in the 1990s recounted how anxieties around 'contamination' led colleagues in other specialisms to stigmatize his work as devalued and shameful:

I think we were talking about why, how we related to the rest of the hospital. I think some people were in, in fear of our patients. People were still worried that they might get infected themselves, we might, we might be contaminated … there were still people who felt a disproportionate amount of resource was being put over to, homosexuals and, black people, and, injecting drug users, are you worthwhile to be treated, invested in, given a special ward, special doctors, special nurses, special pharmacists, what's all that about?[12]

In a 2009 study of HIV stigma in Lesotho, Malawi, South Africa, Swaziland and Tanzania, 83 per cent of nurses had some experience of what the authors term 'stigma events', such as 'people said nurses who provide HIV/AIDS care are HIV positive', or 'someone called a nurse names because she takes care of HIV/AIDS patients'.[13] Healthcare workers engaged in hospital work with SARS patients in East Taiwan also reported 'feeling stigmatized and rejected in their neighbourhood'.[14]

Testimonies from Ugandan nurses providing care in an Ebola outbreak in 2000 and 2001 further illustrate the effects that shame could have on personal relationships:

Our clothes were burned, and our children kept away from us, our families shunned us and were afraid of us. My children would not shake my hand and told me not to ride my bike home (from work) because it might carry Ebola.[15]

Ebola offers an instructive comparison with Covid-19. Particularly after 2014, successive outbreaks attracted significant international attention and were accompanied by the movement of international medical personnel to work in affected areas. While doctors and nurses were subject to localized, relational experiences of avoidance and shame, in their countries of origin and intervention, some also became the subject of a more general panic over contagion in the broader public imaginary of the countries they returned to.[16] Even before she had been repatriated, a Danish nurse recalled seeing hostile comments on Facebook adverts raising money or awareness for Ebola: 'People were commenting, saying "Why do the people need to return and contaminate all of us in Denmark?" and "They should be placed in a camp somewhere for those 3 weeks" and since we were only about 5 people returning, it was, it felt personal to me.'[17]

In circumstances that foreshadowed the shaming experiences of Chris Higgins, Wojciech Rokita and Jean-Robert Ngola, the American physician Dr Craig Spencer was hospitalized with Ebola symptoms in New York after working with patients in Guinea in 2014. His movements and behaviour were painstakingly reconstructed and dissected in detail by national and international newspapers, online and in print, with extensive public conjecture over what he should and shouldn't have done.[18] His case reflected a series of conditions which would later be important contexts for doctor-shaming in Covid-19: long histories of shame and fear around doctors and nurses as potential vectors for disease combined with a fraught and brittle atmosphere of apprehension over contagion. With Spencer's identity as healer visibly and strikingly inverted, the rapid exchange of information and opinion online enabled him – and other healthcare workers – to be shamed in mass participatory events.

In the UK, healthcare workers on the frontline of Covid-19 during 2020 were similarly victims of stigmatization and shaming, sometimes leading to violence and abuse. The primary driver of shame and stigma directed at healthcare workers was related to a fear of contamination, an anxiety that healthcare workers were potential super-spreaders who would breach the virus's confinement within medical spaces and bring it to the community at large. The fear of contamination and of spreading the virus led to many stories regarding the mistreatment of healthcare workers. Care workers were spat at and verbally abused in supermarkets, with accusations of being 'killers' and 'carriers of death'.[19] Several healthcare workers were evicted from their homes by landlords for fear of contagion.[20] Nurses were instructed to hide their ID cards and disguise their uniforms on their way to and from work for fear of physical and verbal abuse.[21] There were material bases for this fear of healthcare workers in the UK in 2020, namely, the lack of adequate testing and widespread shortages of PPE, which affected the UK's ability to respond to Covid-19 and manage its spread, particularly to healthcare workers.

Conversations about PPE dominated the early stages of the pandemic, with widespread shortages in the UK causing substantial concern. So, it is possible that, when members of the public shamed healthcare workers, their response was based on a clearly articulated connection between the workers' lack of protection, their risk of infection and their potential to pass on the virus. More likely, however, these connections were latent: PPE shortages contributed to a total impression of the NHS in a state of crisis, which fed into a general anxiety about healthcare workers. This anxiety was then expressed either through abuse or in acts of solidarity, such as Clap for Carers, or in a general effort to forego medical procedures that weren't directly related to Covid-19. What this doesn't explain is how PPE shortages affected the healthcare workers themselves, and how, quite apart from the *shaming* of healthcare workers, these shortages played a small but important role in their experiences of *shame*.

PPE shortages and the rhetoric of wartime

In a May 2020 survey of nursing staff by the Royal College of Nurses, a third reported some concerns with access to PPE.[22] During the Covid tracker survey by the British Medical Council, concerns about eye protection, facemasks and gowns repeatedly emerged. In the first week of March, 49 per cent of respondents were satisfied with the supplies of gowns, while only 29 per cent and 22 per cent felt secure about the supplies of facemasks and eye protection, respectively.[23] Of the latter, 20 per cent reported having no access to supplies at all. And while these numbers improved over the course of April into May, the residual anxiety about supplies stuck. In Hoernke et al.'s review of frontline healthcare workers feelings about PPE during the pandemic, sourced through a combination of semi-structured interviews, mass media and policy documents, care workers reported problems with guidance and training in PPE use, with the procurement and supply of PPE, and with the barriers PPE set up for the delivery of care.[24] In addition to shortages, inconsistent guidance as to what PPE was required, influenced in part by the lack of supply and in part by rapid developments in understanding the virus, left healthcare workers feeling overwhelmed by guidance from multiple sources. As we go on to suggest, the vulnerability healthcare workers felt provided a fertile ground for feelings of shame to emerge. These feelings, as we discuss below, were exacerbated by the emergence of a wartime rhetoric.

PPE shortages and a paucity of testing contributed to a more general rhetoric of wartime and rationing. This rhetoric, however, was by no means unique to the UK. All across the globe, political and media messages about the Covid-19 crisis were saturated with the language of military violence and conflict. 'We are at war', declared the French president Emmanuel Macron on 16 March.[25] The previous month China's vice-premier Sun Chunlan described China as facing 'wartime conditions', while the Chinese State Media called the public health response to Covid-19 a 'People's War'.[26] On 18 March, Donald Trump referred to himself as a 'wartime president', and shortly afterwards Boris Johnson likened his own administration to a 'wartime government' facing a 'deadly enemy'.[27] Johnson's daily coronavirus meetings were dubbed, internally, the 'war cabinet'.[28] The abundance and insistence on war metaphors in the UK, many argued, was intensified by Boris Johnson's personal fascination with Winston Churchill, with the Covid-19 crisis providing Johnson with the opportunity to position himself as the UK's most recent 'wartime' prime minister.[29]

Taking Johnson's lead, the UK government and media fully embraced the metaphors of wartime, with the repeated invocation of the Second World War, a period that is highly venerated in the British national psyche as demonstrating the exceptionalism and resilience of ordinary British people in the face of significant tragedy and adversity. Comparisons to the Second World War were used liberally as a means to rally the general public in the face of the ongoing Covid-19 crisis, where the British public was repeatedly told to embrace the 'blitz spirit', which refers to the 'keep calm and carry on' stoic attitude that allegedly characterized the British during the war. The 'blitz spirit' was repeatedly invoked by the UK government as a means of rallying the nation to face not only the public health crisis but also the immediate hardships and disruptions that resulted from the nationwide lockdown imposed on 26 March 2020.[30]

The blitz spirit sentiment was institutionalized on 5 April 2020, when the head of state, Elizabeth Windsor, addressed the nation in a special broadcast to acknowledge the hardships the British public was facing during lockdown. Praising the British attributes of 'self-discipline and quiet good-humoured resolve' in the face of adversity, Elizabeth famously ended her address with a brief, spoken excerpt from the chorus of Vera Lynn's famous WWII song 'We'll Meet Again'.[31] Elizabeth's use of the phrase inspired graffiti, placards in shop windows, a patriotic BBC singalong and a billboard display in Piccadilly Circus. While celebrated as morale-boosting in the mainstream media, the sociologist Franziska Kohlt reads this as a deliberate invocation of nostalgia and an elaborate invitation to participate in nationalistic ritual.[32] Indeed, the UK's heavy-handed invocation of Second World War metaphors was by no means unproblematic. As medical semiotician Michael Flexer writes:

> More than any other rhetorical device, over-stretched analogies with the Second World War, already in the ascendant in UK political discourse since 2008, are the lingua franca of COVID-19. This time around, we are simultaneously the besieged of the Blitz in the bomb shelters and the lightning strike Luftwaffe of the Blitzkrieg.[33]

This macho language of confrontation and the inexorable appeal to Second World War kitsch was not merely muddy in its object, as Flexer notes, but also resulted in an insidious process of elision between medical and military interventions, personnel and sacrifice. National figures – such as the Health Secretary Matt Hancock and the Second World War veteran turned fundraiser Captain Tom Moore – played into a conceptual alignment already well-connected in a particular kind of sentimental patriotic imaginary, enabling a loose and easy conflation of 'health care with war and soldiers.'[34]

Indeed, the notion of the 'blitz spirit' is not unproblematic, as the historian Richard Overy notes, where the 'awful realities of being bombed' during the Second World War, including significant experiences of fear, panic, grief and trauma, were 'disguised' with 'tales of British resolve.'[35] The idea of the 'blitz spirit' was invented, Overy argues, to avoid having to acknowledge or address the serious psychological trauma that resulted from wartime experiences such as raids and bombings, using a public insistence on outward expressions of calmness and cheerfulness to minimize the danger and damage that were stark realities of the war.[36] An insistence on the blitz spirit, as a desirable attitude to take during the Covid-19 crisis, set up problematic expectations, not only for ordinary citizens but especially for healthcare workers, who were expected to just 'keep calm and carry on', even in the face of significant stress, grief, overwork and burnout, within hospitals that were ill-equipped to ensure their basic physical safety. As a result, complaining, quitting and not coping were signs of weakness and cowardliness and, hence, occasions for shame.

By March 2020, the NHS had been subsumed by military metaphors. Health workers were 'servicemen' on the 'frontline' 'battling' 'an invisible enemy'.[37] This metaphoric landscape served as a means to make sense of the gruelling conditions that NHS workers found themselves in. There was a sense of emergency, with ICU wards overflowing, a relentless onslaught of very sick patients, high death rates and limited treatment options, all underpinned by a widespread fear of infection or contamination. The metaphors of wartime resonated strongly not only with healthcare workers but also the general population who were living in unprecedented peacetime conditions, ordered to 'stay at home' in order to 'save lives'. Lockdown restrictions had many striking parallels with the conditions of wartime such as occupations, or restrictions because of bombings and other military attacks. The UK's first national Covid-19 lockdown involved limited access to commodities and services, effectively proscribed all but local travel and imposed extraordinary boundaries on personal freedoms, social and romantic behaviour, and the use of public space.

War metaphors are compelling because they appeal to basic and widely shared schematic knowledge, expressing a sense of emergency that captures attention and motivates action, while also justifying extreme living or working conditions where individuals may have to make uncharacteristic sacrifices.[38] Questioning whether 'we really want a war on Aids', Judith Wilson Ross made the important point that 'the metaphor gives us an opportunity to injure without having to admit that is what we are doing. In war, much is excused that would not be tolerated in peace-time. In the press of war, we do not have time for niceties.'[39] As Ross makes clear, the use of war metaphors in public health, medicine, and epidemic or pandemic contexts is not new. The poet John Donne referred to his experience of illness as 'a siege', and medical men such as Thomas Sydenham related disease to battle in the seventeenth century, and perhaps earlier.[40] This tendency gathered frequency in nineteenth-century bacteriology, with the register of war and conflict attached to microbes and bacteria as a means to imagine the otherwise invisible 'threat' that viruses and bacteria pose to the human body. Louis Pasteur, for example, described viruses in 'a language of invading armies laying siege to the body that becomes a battlefield'.[41]

Increasingly co-opted for a range of complex and intractable medical problems from dementia to cancer, military metaphors offer a usable cultural script for global leaders engaged in particularly visible and high-profile biopolitics. As such, they have always performed specific political work, including around the deflection and attribution of shame.[42] Susan Sontag's pioneering work on cancer explored how the language of war led to feelings of shame and dehumanization among patients, a problem with a long and enduring legacy.[43] Assigning a belligerent anthropomorphic identity to illness or disease can also fulfil the function of rendering it 'aggressive' or difficult to predict; legitimate critique of prevention and control measures, for example, is effectively de-fanged by the militarized imagery of sacrifice and defence. War metaphors also carry the convenient implication of armistice, an identifiable and singular end, with little basis in either military or epidemiological histories.[44] As Chapter 6 of this volume explores, nationalistic modes of thinking about health also rely on scripts which often crowd out necessary languages of international cooperation.

The direct implications of wartime rhetoric for healthcare workers in the UK were profoundly ambivalent. On the one hand, there was a public outpouring of support for those 'fighting' on the 'frontline'. Clap for Carers was established and healthcare workers were routinely cast as 'heroes', 'angels' and the 'tirelessly dedicated'.[45] Frontline healthcare workers were applauded and honoured for their hard work and sacrifice, for tirelessly 'battling' against the 'enemy'. One Mass Observation testimony explored the mythos around their contribution, and the affective resonance it had on the responder:

> On Thursday evenings when the NHS clap takes place for example, I always have a lump in my throat and a very solemn feeling of helplessness and perhaps even guilt. Due to being so content with my home life at the moment that does often lead to many twangs of guilt knowing that others are risking their lives everyday either helping self-lives or fighting disease.[46]

This sentiment of personal appreciation by an individual citizen reached its pinnacle when Elizabeth Windsor awarded the George's Cross, Britain's highest award for gallantry and heroism, to the NHS in July 2021. Citing the 'courage, compassion and dedication' of NHS staff, especially in 'recent times', Elizabeth institutionalized the militarized lionization of healthcare workers.[47]

On the other hand, however, these sorts of gestures were viewed by many as 'disingenuous', particularly when 'the appreciation' did not lead to 'real action' to 'improve working conditions'.[48] Further, heroic status was double edged, and brought its own potential stigma and shame. Cast as 'soldiers' in a 'war', NHS workers were expected to make personal sacrifices. In fact, they were expected to put their own lives on the line, working without adequate PPE or testing, and often lambasted if they refused to do so. In an NHS that was already under considerable strain due to chronic underfunding, doctors and other healthcare workers were expected to work gruelling shifts without adequate staffing, resources, support and, crucially, PPE. As a University of Bath large-scale qualitative research study into the experience of frontline doctors during Covid-19 revealed, doctors felt they were working at '100% capacity, 100% of the time', while feeling 'expendable', 'exposed' and 'unprotected', left traumatized by the lack of support from the government. As one doctor expressed: 'I'm not a COVID hero, I'm COVID cannon fodder'.[49] Central to these experiences was significant emotional strain, with exhaustion, grief, stress and burnout being commonly reported.[50] Of course, shame was part of this landscape of emotions. Not only were doctors actively subject to pandemic shaming, with reports of doctors being 'bullied and shamed' into treating patients with Covid-19 when lacking adequate PPE,[51] but there were also significant accounts of healthcare workers feeling shame when being unable, or feeling unable, to 'serve' on the 'frontline'. An early critique of the lionization of health workers during Covid-19 put the problem as follows: 'The opposite of a hero is a coward, or a deserter. There have been reports of health professionals feeling "ashamed" for choosing not to "go to war". Alarmingly, some third-year nurses have been reported being abused or publicly shamed on Twitter for not taking up an offer to register early to "fight" COVID-19'.[52]

This polarized treatment of NHS workers, as the recipients of both applause and abuse, is not so contradictory as it first appears. As the philosopher Richard Kearney notes, a tendency to 'othering', to create 'gods' and 'monsters' out of our peers, occurs most readily in times of 'terror or war'.[53] Many of us in the UK experienced the early days of the Covid-19 crisis remotely, through an affective landscape consisting of both a generalized anxiety, in the face of an invisible and potentially deadly 'enemy' against which most of us could do nothing, and a diffused hope, in the anticipation of those on the 'frontline' 'defeating' the 'enemy'. Hence, the simultaneous valorizing and shunning of healthcare workers can be understood as an attempt to find both scapegoats to blame (to assuage fear and uncertainty) and heroes to lionize (to amplify hope). Both scapegoating and lionization landed on NHS workers, rendering them both more, and less, than human. They were positioned as potential enemies (exacerbating the crisis by spreading the disease or by being 'cowards' who shunned their 'duty'), and as heroes (saving us from the crisis by eliminating the disease).

Referencing ancient myths and contemporary terrorism, Kearney observes how common this pattern of dual 'othering' becomes in times of war and terror: 'in our confusion, we have been known to turn the Other into a monster *and* a god'.[54] If the *shaming* of healthcare workers may be explained by the othering processes of wartime rhetoric, this does not quite explain how we link this rhetoric to healthcare workers' expressions of vulnerability and their confessions of *feeling shame*.

In general, doctors and other healthcare workers are particularly vulnerable to shame and shaming. Issues which directly affect a doctor's ability to deliver healthcare effectively, including long working hours, staff shortages, bed shortages, waiting lists and limited treatment options, can be perceived as shortcomings in an individual's performance, rather than part of wider systemic problems. In addition, our cultural expectations regarding doctors are that they are infallible and superhuman; they must make flawless diagnosis and treatment decisions, leaving no room for doubt, error or imperfection. In addition, they must not be physically or emotionally vulnerable: they should not get sick, need to sleep on a shift, have mental health problems or have other personal needs while treating others. The overwhelming negative public response to cases where doctors have made mistakes, or are *perceived* to have made mistakes, suggests that this expectation of infallibility and invulnerability exacerbates feelings of violated trust. We are outraged when doctors fail us by being human.

These expectations create a situation where doctors find themselves in a situation curiously parallel to that given by Judith Butler in her discussion of the sovereign subject, a position which 'not only denies its own constitutive injurability but tries to relocate injurability in the other'.[55] This position is emphasized by treating an other already marked by injury, the patient. Such responses, the philosopher Bonnie Mann has argued, are often strongly gendered, even when its protagonists do not present as men: it results in a 'sovereign masculinity' characterized by 'a denial of both physical and intersubjective vulnerability'.[56] But sovereign masculinity does not simply emerge as an ideal out of nowhere. 'It must be produced', Mann writes, observing too that 'shame always accompanies sovereign masculinity because it plays a central part in its production. This is why we see systematic, relentless, repetitious shaming, wherever sovereign masculinity is the aspirational ideal'.[57] Mann turns to the shaming and hazing practices that characterize the training of military personnel. Through repeated acts of shaming, personnel are expected to deny and reject their own feelings of vulnerability, thus transforming feelings of shame into feelings of power. Mann calls this transformation a 'shame-to-power conversion'.[58]

Ongoing studies of medical education have shown the ubiquity of shaming practices and shame experiences amongst medical students.[59] Although it is tendentious to claim that such practices are meant to create a shame-to-power conversion, as described by Mann, we might say that the militarized rhetoric of the pandemic brought medicalized sovereign subjectivity into closer alignment with Mann's notion of sovereign masculinity. This may account for why war metaphors produced such feelings of shame in healthcare workers unwilling to deny their own vulnerabilities.

Of course, the most significant harm of the war metaphor was not shame but positioning NHS workers as expendable; they became an inevitable cost of wartime: soldiers die in battle; that is the price of 'waging a war'. Between March and December 2020, 850 healthcare workers in the UK died of Covid-19, many of them from ethnic minority backgrounds.[60] With healthcare workers subject to painful experiences of public shaming and exposure, doctors, nurses and support staff from racialized groups were placed under particular forms of strain. The embodied product of institutional racism, historic health inequalities among populations designated as 'BAME' meant that people of colour formed the majority of early deaths among healthcare workers, a crucial factor in the broader realization that Covid-19 has a disproportionate effect on members of minoritized communities.[61] Structural racism within the NHS also meant that 'BAME' healthcare workers felt unduly pressured to work in unsafe conditions, and less able to advocate for adequate PPE.[62]

The following chapter explores how the Covid-19 pandemic was allowed to exacerbate and reproduce pre-existing health inequalities and experiences of chronic shame. It situates the anti-Asian racism of the early pandemic in a longer historical context of colonialist anxieties over conspiracies and contamination, and addresses the role of shame in both overt racist violence and structural systems of marginalization and oppression. Analysing systemic communication failures over the impact of Covid-19 on 'BAME' populations, it suggests that attempts to deflect shame away from the institutions and processes that perpetuate racism made undue room for shame among its victims, further worsening health inequalities characterized by long experiences of political and medical shaming.

Notes

1. Merran Hitchick, '"Flabbergasted": Melbourne Doctor with Coronavirus Symptoms Continued Seeing Patients', *The Guardian*, 00:48 BST, 7 March 2020. https://www.theguardian.com/world/2020/mar/07/flabbergasted-melbourne-doctor-with-coronavirus-symptoms-continued-seeing-patients.

2. Call Wahlquist, 'Doctor Who Had Coronavirus Demands Apology from Victorian Health Minister over 'Inaccuracies', *The Guardian*, 00:09 GMT, 8 March 2020. https://www.theguardian.com/world/2020/mar/08/doctor-who-had-coronavirus-demands-apology-from-victorian-health-minister-over-inaccuracies.

3. Luna Dolezal and Arthur Rose, 'Naming and Shaming: Covid-19 and the Health Professional', *BMJ Medical Humanities Blog*, 7 April 2020. https://blogs.bmj.com/medical-humanities/2020/04/07/naming-and-shaming-covid-19-and-the-medical-professional/.

4. Luna Dolezal, Arthur Rose and Fred Cooper, 'COVID-19, Online Shaming and Healthcare Professionals', *The Lancet* vol. 389 (2021), 482–83.

5. D. T. Max, 'The Public-Shaming Pandemic', *The New Yorker*, 21 September 2020.

6. Diana Duong, 'Does Shaming Have a Place in Public Health?', *CMAJ News*, 11 December 2020. https://cmajnews.com/2020/12/11/shaming-1095910/.

7. Mark Earnest, 'On Becoming a Plague Doctor', *New England Journal of Medicine* vol. 383:e64 (2020). https://doi.org/10.1056/NEJMp2011418.

8. Rebecca Rideal, 'What Were Women's Lives Like during the 17th-century Plague?', *History Extra*, 10 January 2022. https://www.historyextra.com/period/stuart/women-of-the-plague/.

9. Samuel Kline Cohn, 'Cholera Revolts: A Class Struggle We May Not Like', *Social History* vol. 42:2 (2017), 162–80. https://doi.org/10.1080/03071022.2017.1290365.

10. Sean Burrell and Geoffrey Gill, 'The Liverpool Cholera Epidemic of 1832 and Anatomical Dissection–Medical Mistrust and Civil Unrest', *Journal of the History of Medicine and Allied Sciences* vol. 60:4 (2005), 478–98. https://doi.org/10.1093/jhmas/jri061.

11. Samuel K. Cohn Jr, *Epidemics: Hate and Compassion from the Plague of Athens to AIDS* (Oxford: Oxford University Press, 2018), 206–7, 214, 239.

12. Testimony of Simon Barton, HIV Consultant, 'Health Care Workers in HIV: An Oral History in the UK AIDS Era', 5 June 2019. https://www.healthcareworkersinhiv.org.uk/interview-themes/responses-and-attitudes/responses-and-attitudes.

13. William L. Holzemer et al., 'Measuring HIV Stigma for PLHAs and Nurses over Time in Five African Countries', *SAHARA J: Journal of Social Aspects of*

HIV/AIDS Research Alliance vol. 6:2 (2009), 76–82, 78, 81. https://doi.org/10.1 080/17290376.2009.9724933.

14. YaMei Bai et al., 'Survey of Stress Reactions among Health Care Workers Involved with the SARS Outbreak', *Psychiatric Services* vol. 55:9 (2004), 1055–7, 1057. https://doi.org/10.1176/appi.ps.55.9.1055.

15. Bonnie L. Hewlett and Barry S. Hewlett, 'Providing Care and Facing Death: Nursing during Ebola Outbreaks in Central Africa', *Journal of Transcultural Nursing* vol. 16:4 (October 2005), 289–97, 295, 295. https://doi. org/10.1177/1043659605278935.

16. Misse Wester and Johan Giesecke, 'Ebola and Healthcare Worker Stigma', *Scandinavian Journal of Public Health* vol. 47:2 (2019), 99–104. https://doi. org/10.1177/1403494817753450.

17. Stephanie Gee and Morten Skovdal, 'Public Discourses of Ebola Contagion and Courtesy Stigma: The Real Risk to International Health Care Workers Returning Home from the West Africa Ebola Outbreak?', *Qualitative Health Research* vol. 28:9 (July 2018), 1499–508, 1504. https://doi. org/10.1177/1049732318759936.

18. Craig Spencer, 'Having and Fighting Ebola – Public Health Lessons from a Clinician Turned Patient', *New England Journal of Medicine* vol. 372 (2015), 1089–91. https://doi.org/10.1056/NEJMp1501355.

19. Angeline Albert, 'Care Workers Hide Uniforms after Being Spat at and Called "carriers of death,"' *Homecare.co.uk* vol. 13:14 GMT, 7 April 2020. https:// www.homecare.co.uk/news/article.cfm/id/1624098/Care-workers-battling-coronavirus-are-spat-at-in-street-and-called-carriers-of-death.

20. Hannah Mays, 'NHS Paramedic Evicted from Home for Fear He Would Spread COVID-19', *The Guardian* 16:58 GMT, 22 March 2020. https://www. theguardian.com/world/2020/mar/22/nhs-paramedic-evicted-from-home-for-fear-he-would-spread-covid-19?CMP=Share_iOSApp_Other; Sunita Patel-Carstairs, 'Coronavirus: NHS Doctor "evicted from home due to landladies fears over COVID-19"', *Sky News*, 13:26 GMT, 26 March 2020. https://news. sky.com/story/coronavirus-nhs-doctor-evicted-from-home-due-to-landladys-fears-over-covid-19-11963799; Chiara Giordano, 'Coronavirus: NHS Doctor Kicked out by Landlord because of COVID-19 Fears', *The Independent* 17:39 GMT, 25 April 2020. https://www.independent.co.uk/news/health/coronavirus-latest-nhs-doctor-evicted-covid-19-oxford-a9425166.html.

21. Ewan Summerville, 'NHS Nurses Told Not to Wear Uniform Outside of Hospitals after Being Called "Virus Spreaders"', *The Evening Standard*, 28 March 2020. https://www.standard.co.uk/news/uk/coronavirus-nhs-nurses-lewisham-hospital-greenwich-a4400586.html.

22. Royal College of Nursing, 'Second Personal Protective Equipment Survey of UK Nursing Staff Report: Use and Availability of PPE during the COVID-19 Pandemic', Royal College of Nursing, 2020. https://www.rcn.org.uk/-/media/ royal-college-of-nursing/documents/publications/2020/may/009-269.pdf?la=en.

23. British Medical Association, 'Covid Tracker Surveys: Analysing the Impact of Coronavirus on Doctors', https://www.bma.org.uk/advice-and-support/covid-19/what-the-bma-is-doing/covid-19-analysing-the-impact-of-coronavirus-on-doctors.

24. Katarina Hoernke, Nehla Djellouli, Lily Andrews, Sasha Lewis-Jackson, Louisa Manby, Sam Martin, Samantha Vanderslott and Cecilia Vindrola-Padros, 'Frontline Healthcare Workers' Experiences with Personal Protective Equipment during the COVID-19 Pandemic in the UK: A Rapid Qualitative Appraisal', *BMJ open* vol. 11:1, e046199. 20 Jan. 2021. doi:10.1136/bmjopen-2020-046199.

25. Michael Saft, 'From Unknown Virus to Global Crisis: Timeline', *The Guardian* 14 December 2020. https://www.theguardian.com/world/ng-interactive/2020/dec/14/coronavirus-2020-timeline-covid-19.

26. Luke Shors, 'Waging Another Public Health "War"?' *Think Global Health*, 26 February 2020. https://www.thinkglobalhealth.org/article/waging-another-public-health-war.

27. Francesca Panzeri, Simona Di Paola and Filippo Domaneschi, 'Does the COVID-19 War Metaphor Influence Reasoning?', *PLOS ONE* vol. 16:4 (2021), e0250651. https://doi.org/10.1371/journal.pone.0250651.

28. Rebecca Speare-Cole, 'Boris Johnson "raring to go" as he hosts Coronavirus "war cabinet" amid Questions over Government's Strategy', *Evening Standard*, 27 April 2020. https://www.standard.co.uk/news/uk/boris-johnson-back-to-work-coronavirus-meeting-lockdown-a4424566.html.

29. Dawn Foster, 'Boris Johnson's Contradictory Coronavirus Response Is Cowardly and Will Result in Mass Deaths', *Jacobin* 24 March 2020. https://jacobinmag.com/2020/03/boris-johnson-coronavirus-winston-churchill-britain-nhs.

30. Helen Lewis, 'The Spirit of the Blitz', *The Economist*, 21 March 2020. https://www.economist.com/britain/2020/03/21/spirit-of-the-blitz.

31. '"We will meet again": The Queen's Coronavirus Broadcast', *BBC*, 5 April 2020. video, https://www.youtube.com/watch?v=2klmuggOElE.

32. Franziska Kohlt '"Over by Christmas": The Impact of War-metaphors and Other Science-religion Narratives on Science Communication Environments during the Covid-19 Crisis', *SocArXiv*, 10 November 2020. doi:10.31235/osf.io/z5s6a, 6.

33. Michael J. Flexer, 'Having a Moment: The Revolutionary Semiotic of COVID-19', *Wellcome Open Research* vol. 5:134 (2020). https://doi.org/10.12688/wellcomeopenres.15972.1, 6.

34. Kohlt, 'Over by Christmas', 10.

35. Richard Overy, 'Why the Cruel Myth of the "blitz spirit" Is No Model for how to Fight Coronavirus', *The Guardian* 14:37 GMT, 19 March 2020. https://www.theguardian.com/commentisfree/2020/mar/19/myth-blitz-spirit-model-coronavirus.

36. Overy, 'Why the Cruel Myth of the "blitz spirit" Is No Model for How to Fight Coronavirus'.

37. Arthur Rose and Luna Dolezal, 'Stigma and the Logics of Wartime', *Society for Cultural Anthropology*, 5 May 2020. https://culanth.org/fieldsights/stigma-and-the-logics-of-wartime.

38. Stephen J. Flusberg, Teenie Matlock, and Paul H. Thibodeau, 'War Metaphors in Public Discourse', *Metaphor and Symbol* 33, 1 (2018): 1–18.

39. Judith Wilson Ross, 'The Militarization of Disease: Do We Really Want a War on Aids?', *Soundings: An Interdisciplinary Journal* vol. 72:1 (Spring 1989), 39–58, 55.

40. Heather Patricia Lane et al., 'The War against Dementia: Are We Battle Weary Yet?', *Age and Ageing* vol. 42:3 (2013), 281–3. https://doi.org/10.1093/ageing/aft011.

41. Alan Bleakley, 'Force and Presence in the World of Medicine', *Healthcare* vol. 5:58 (2017), 1–8, 4. https://doi.org/10.3390/healthcare5030058.

42. Eunice Castro Seixas, 'War Metaphors in Political Communication on Covid-19', *Frontiers in Sociology*, 25 January 2021. https://doi.org/10.3389/fsoc.2020.583680.

43. Susan Sontag, *Illness as Metaphor* (New York: Farrar, Straus, and Giroux, 1978); Rose K. Hendricks et al., 'Emotional Implications of Metaphor: Consequences of Metaphor Framing for Mindset about Cancer', *Metaphor and Symbol* 33:4 (2018), 267–79. https://doi.org/10.1080/10926488.2018.1549835.

44. Dora Vargha and Jeremy A. Greene, 'How Epidemics End', *Boston Review*, 30 June 2020. https://bostonreview.net/articles/jeremy-greene-dora-vargha-how-epidemics-end-or-dont/.

45. Rose and Dolezal, 'Stigma and the Logics of Wartime'.

46. Mass Observation Archive (University of Sussex): Replies to 2020 Special Directive [C7485].

47. Caroline Davies, 'The Queen Awards George Cross to NHS Mark 70 Years of Public Service', *The Guardian*, 00:01 BST, 5 July 2021. https://www.theguardian.com/society/2021/jul/05/queen-awards-george-cross-to-nhs-to-mark-70-years-of-public-service.

48. Elaine L. Kinsella and Rachel C. Summer, 'High Ideas: The Misappropriation and Reappropriation of the Heroic Label in the midst of a Global Pandemic', *Journal of Medical Ethics*, Epub ahead of print (2021). doi:10.1136/medethics-2021-107236.

49. Sophie Harris, Elizabeth Jenkinson, Edward Carlton, Tom Roberts and Jo Daniels, '"It's Been Ugly": A Large-Scale Qualitative Study into the Difficulties Frontline Doctors Faced across Two Waves of the COVID-19 Pandemic', *International Journal of Environmental Research and Public Health* vol. 18:24 (2021), 13067. https://doi.org/10.3390/ijerph182413067.

50. Rachel C. Summer and Elaine L. Kinsella, "'It's Like a Kick in the Teeth": The Emergence of Novel Predictors of Burnout in Frontline Workers during Covid-19', *Frontiers in Psychology* vol. 12 (2021), 645504.

51. Denis Campbell, 'Doctors Lacking PPE "bullied" into Treating Covid-19 Patients', *The Guardian*, 00:00 BST, 7 April 2020, https://www.theguardian.com/world/2020/apr/06/nhs-doctors-lacking-ppe-bullied-into-treating-covid-19-patients.

52. Ruth Naughton-Doe, 'Going to War, or Going to Work?', *Nursing Times*, 14 May 2020. https://www.nursingtimes.net/opinion/going-to-war-or-going-to-work-14-05-2020/.

53. Richard Kearney, *Strangers, Gods and Monsters: Interpreting Otherness* (London: Routledge, 2002), 4.

54. Kearney, *Strangers, Gods and Monsters*, 5.

55. Judith Butler, *Frames of War: When Is Life Grievable?* (London: Verso Books, 2009), 278.

56. Bonnie Mann, *Sovereign Masculinity: Gender Lessons from the War on Terror* (Oxford: Oxford University Press, 2014), 109.

57. Mann, *Sovereign Masculinity*, 109.

58. Mann, *Sovereign Masculinity*, 124.

59. Arthur Rose, 'Shame-to-cynicism Conversion in *The Citadel* and *The House of God*', *Medical Humanities*, Vol. 47:2 (2021), 219.

60. David Berger, 'Up the Line to Death: Covid-19 Has Revealed a Mortal Betrayal of the World's Healthcare Workers', *The BMJ Opinion*, 29 January 2021. https://blogs.bmj.com/bmj/2021/01/29/up-the-line-to-death-covid-19-has-revealed-a-mortal-betrayal-of-the-worlds-healthcare-workers/.

61. British Medical Association, 'COVID-19: The Risk to BAME Doctors', 24 August 2021. https://www.bma.org.uk/advice-and-support/covid-19/your-health/covid-19-the-risk-to-bame-doctors.

62. Keith Cooper, 'BAME Doctors Hit Worse by Lack of PPE', *British Medical Association*, 24 April 2020. https://www.bma.org.uk/news-and-opinion/bame-doctors-hit-worse-by-lack-of-ppe.

CHAPTER 3
COUGHING WHILE ASIAN: SHAME AND RACIALIZED BODIES

---

3 February 2020. Tow-Arboleda Films uploads a short film titled 'Coughing While Asian Corona Virus' to YouTube. It follows an Asian man, played by Michael Tow, affecting a cough to comic effect. The opening scene establishes the phenomenon: Tow coughs briefly at the gym during a Covid-19 news bulletin; the woman using the equipment beside him quickly leaves, her eyes wide with alarm. Bemused, Tow gingerly sniffs one armpit, wondering whether she was driven away by his body odour. Tow's character begins to deploy his cough to minor advantage: he uses it to disperse the queue at a coffee shop, then alarms his co-workers in a packed lift. The final scene sees him settle uncomfortably in a crowded cinema. As he raises his fist towards his mouth, he is startled by a long, hacking cough. The other filmgoers flee in panic. The camera pans around to a young Asian woman, wearing a face mask, who winks knowingly at Tow.

The film is funny, and clearly intended to be so. The overarching joke pivots on the subversion of and resistance to shame and discrimination, as the two Asian characters exploit the ignorance and prejudice around them. Rather than feeling shamed or diminished by racist anxieties over contamination, they use their coughs, shamelessly, to get what they want. This narrative device draws attention to the exaggerated responses of the other characters, illustrating the stigma attached to social avoidance. As the accompanying text makes clear, the filmmakers aimed to provide a comedic response to a serious problem:

> Asians and Asian Americans are getting targeted and bullied, as anti Asian rhetoric sweeps the land and media as a response to the Corona Virus. All over the news, reports of Asians, particularly Chinese, are being mentally and physically abused. An Asian male in Australia died

of a heart attack when bystanders wouldn't come to his aid because they falsely were afraid he had the corona virus.[1]

Like Lauren Aratini's *Guardian* article of the same name, 'coughing while Asian' invoked a specific linguistic script on racist or heteronormative surveillance and discipline, contrasting innocent or unremarkable behaviour with an over-policed and marginalized identity.[2] Examples with longer histories include 'driving while black' and 'walking while trans', both references to police profiling and state violence in the United States.[3] In the early phase of the pandemic, we saw a parallel effort to inflame and encourage verbal and physical abuse towards Asians in the United States, with President Donald Trump's frequent pronouncements on the 'China Virus' and the 'Wuhan Virus', and his derogatory use of the term 'Kung Flu' in June 2020.[4] Although the UK government has publicly condemned overt instances of racist violence and humiliation, a Conservative council leader who attributed the emergence of the virus to 'somebody eating undercooked bat soup' was found not to have breached his code of conduct.[5]

In this chapter, we explore how practices of racialized shaming and scapegoating emerged in the UK during 2020, following well-worn patterns of stigma, marginalization and exclusion.[6] Following the initial shaming hyper-visibility of individuals assumed to be of Chinese origin in the first months of the pandemic, we trace how the public health interventions of summer, autumn and winter 2020, such as local lockdowns and tier systems, led to the shaming and blaming of ethnic minorities. Politicians developed a racialized preoccupation with intergenerational households and religious observance, which they implicated in emerging data on increased morbidity and mortality among people placed in the now-discarded Black Asian and Minority Ethnic (BAME) demographic category. Even while medical and academic conversations about structural racism, social deprivation and health inequalities surrounded disparities in Covid-19 mortality rates, the acknowledgement of structural disadvantage in relation to health outcomes was overshadowed by discourses which directed blame for infection and illness towards individuals and communities. Exploring the intersections between public health policy, racism, structural inequalities and experiences of shame, this chapter explores how public health interventions which mobilized shame exacerbated existing inequalities, particularly along lines of race and ethnicity.

'I don't want your coronavirus in my country!'

Initiating a debate on anti-Asian racism in the House of Commons in October 2020, the Labour MP for Luton North, Sarah Owen, described a handful of the hundreds of hate crimes which had been reported in the preceding months:

> In March, Jonathan Mok, a 23-year-old student from Singapore, was punched and kicked in the face on Oxford Street by a group of men. He heard shouts of 'Coronavirus!' and was told, 'I don't want your coronavirus in my country!' British-Chinese filmmaker Lucy Sheen was on her way to rehearsals on a bus, when a white male passenger whispered in her ear – forgive me for the unparliamentary language: 'Why don't you f-off back to China and take your filth with you?' In Hitchin, just down the road from my constituency, a takeaway owner was spat at and repeatedly asked if he had coronavirus.[7]

Incidents such as these led to feelings of hyper-visibility and fears over potential confrontation and shame. As one Mass Observation correspondent put it, 'I feel very Asian in public'.[8] Her anxieties as a racialized woman in the UK were fuelled by the many anti-Chinese racist attacks reported in the national and international news. Heightened public scrutiny for 'looking Chinese' corresponded to an attribution of contamination, infection and blame for the virus. 'Coronavirus', Owen added, 'has been given the face of a Chinese Asian person'.[9]

A conversation between two academics at the University of Edinburgh, Nini Fang and Shan-Jan Sarah Liu, on 'being Yellow women in the time of COVID-19', details the pernicious effects of anxiety over (and experiences of) harassment and social shaming. Liu spoke about her terror of unwanted scrutiny and attention, and competing demands for her physical and emotional safety, such as not wanting to wear a mask for fear of standing out and not wanting to leave the house despite the well-known benefit to mental health. Freedom from trepidation over confrontation or abuse, she explained, 'was a white privilege I didn't have. Eventually, when I did finally go into my office to collect things, I got spat at'. For Fang, pandemic racism created an uncomfortable reliance on her partner in public spaces; attending an online seminar, she was humiliated and shamed while asking a question of the speaker. 'Was this social shaming partly stoked by the pandemic', she speculated, 'which has been racialized as the disease of the East?'[10]

Anti-Asian racism during Covid-19 is a multi-layered and complex phenomenon, tapping into long histories of anti-Chinese sentiment in the UK and elsewhere, particularly relating to infectious disease. In the context of Covid-19, deeper suspicions of global mobility and migration were collapsed into accusations of transmission and contamination. Developing long-established orientalist tropes, this racist scrutiny combined contradictory narratives on the origins of the virus. In one imagining, unclean or unsavoury eating habits had resulted in the transmission of the virus from bats (or sometimes pangolins) to humans; in the other, the Chinese government had released the virus, by mistake or intent, as part of a programme of ongoing efforts to manipulate, destabilize and subjugate the global West.[11]

Incidents of racist violence during Covid-19 were encouraged and exacerbated by a proliferation of online racism in the form of hate speech, anti-Asian memes, images, videos and cartoons, and conspiracy theories.[12] The overall intention was to blame, shame and degrade individuals and communities, implicating victims (and members of East Asian and Southeast Asian communities in general) as dirty or unhygienic spreaders of contagion. In predominantly white nations and communities, racist language and violence have always been methods of policing white supremacy, of communicating to ethnic minorities that hard-won civil rights and safeties are fragile and easily set aside. They have always been about degradation, humiliation and shame.

Shame is a common response to racism, where the feeling arises not because someone has done something wrong, or necessarily feels flawed or at fault in some way; instead, racism-induced shame is intimately related to social power.[13] As the philosopher Aness Webster notes, shame arises because an individual experiences a 'loss of power over when her stigmatised racialised identity is made salient'.[14] A common harm of racism, she argues, is the 'emotional cost of feeling shame … and an ongoing vulnerability to shame'.[15] In this way, racist violence and verbal abuse frequently result in shame, fear and insecurity, not just for direct victims but for members of the targeted group as a whole. The taunts that Mok and the takeaway owner endured rehearsed well-travelled cultural tropes over migration and contagion, brought out even more forcefully in the whispered invective to Sheen. The reference to 'filth' collapsed fears over viral transmission with racist intimations of dirtiness and poor hygiene, keying into widespread speculation and scapegoating over the origins of the virus in a Wuhan wet market.

Indeed, one of the more publicized examples in the early pandemic was the case of 'Bat Soup Girl'. *Russia Today* and *The Daily Mail* found footage of a Chinese woman eating a bat, publicizing it as 'disturbing' and 'revolting' evidence of eating habits in Wuhan.[16] As the video gained traction, the woman, travel vlogger Wang Mengyun, came forward to apologize for eating the bat. Explaining that the video was filmed as part of a travel segment on Palau, Micronesia, in 2017, she detailed the online abuse she had received, including phrases like 'You're abnormal' and 'You're disgusting'. Although Wang was undoubtedly the direct victim of the abuse, commentators like James Palmer have noted how 'the Palau video has been deployed in the United States and Europe to renew an old narrative about the supposedly disgusting eating habits of foreigners'.[17] Despite working from incompatible theories, narratives on the genesis of Covid-19 in Wuhan wet market or secret government laboratory share a consistent internal logic, drawing a clear conceptual line between a healthy and hygienic West and a polluting and infectious East, with disease 'coded as a foreign invasion'.[18]

There is a serious historical question playing counterpoint to these shaming causative stories. What is historically specific about anti-Chinese racism in the UK, and the way it relates to contagion, conspiracy and shame? As an extensive literature of scholarship attests, real or manufactured anxieties over disease have long been a feature of anti-immigration rhetoric in the global West.[19] With both the UK government and the Opposition attempting to outdo one another on border policing as a technique of virus management, imagined dichotomies between a healthy polity and a diseased and dangerous other are very much here to stay.[20]

When Sarah Owen spoke in parliament on anti-Asian racism, she criticized the Metropolitan Police's continued use of the term 'oriental people': 'we do not have enough time in this debate to unpack what is wrong with that term, but it is 2020, not 1920'.[21] Owen's reference to 1920 was astute, gesturing to particularly pervasive patterns of anti-Chinese racism around the turn of – and well into – the twentieth century. Anti-Semitic and Sinophobic propaganda framed Jewish and Chinese migrants as 'carriers of "foreign" diseases', a characterization rooted in a visceral and shaming language of illness and dirt. The pamphleteer Joseph Banister, for example, intentionally blurred the boundaries between the two, describing Jews as an 'Asiatic' and 'Oriental' presence whose blood was 'loaded with scrofula'.[22] In his 2020 essay on 'The Chinese Virus', Roger

Luckhurst explores the Gothic literary traditions that drew from and fed into political anxieties over Eastern contagion in the nineteenth and early twentieth centuries, including fictional depictions of exotic plagues ravaging Britain, allegorical writing on vampirism (with identical tropes of infection and pollution) and literatures preoccupied with Chinese and Japanese expansionism.[23] Other contemporaries tapped into an overlapping characterization of Chinese migrants and nationals as insidious conspirators and 'puppet masters', degrading and debauching Western society from within. The General Secretary of the National Union of Dock Labourers, for example, warned in 1906 that the Chinese labourer 'comes here like an international octopus spreading its tentacles everywhere'.[24] Although carrying no obvious connotations of dirt and disease, the imagery of the octopus is relatively easy to parse: fluid, alien, manipulative, strangling and impossible to pin down.[25]

After 1913, Sax Rohmer's famous supervillain, Dr Fu Manchu, simultaneously drew on and sustained the racialized image of shadowy and malevolent criminal networks, and evil masterminds bent on world domination.[26] As Luckhurst puts it, Manchu is tentacular, 'always slithering his arms around Western interests'.[27] In the first of Rohmer's prolific canon, *The Mystery of Dr. Fu Manchu* (published in the United States as *The Insidious Dr. Fu Manchu*), the antagonist reveals himself as an expert in the deadly application of animal and biological agents:

'One of my pets, Mr. Smith,' he said, suddenly opening his eyes fully so that they blazed like green lamps. 'I have others, equally useful. My scorpions – have you met my scorpions? No? My pythons and hamadryads? Then there are my fungi and my tiny allies, the bacilli. I have a collection in my laboratory quite unique. Have you ever visited Molokai, the leper island, Doctor? No?'[28]

In this striking passage, Chinese culpability for the spread of disease is reconfigured – not as a concomitant of poor hygiene and dirtiness, or even an innate racial affliction, but as an esoteric and deliberate biological weapon. Manchu's reference to the leper colony on the Hawaiian island Moloka'i played into widespread beliefs that Hansen's disease had been introduced to Hawaii by Chinese immigrants in the 1830s and 1840s, in the context of wider associations between the disease and Chinese migration.[29] Given Manchu's unnaturally long life and professed mastery over bacterial technologies, this reads as a boast as well as a threat. A later iteration of the arch-villain (in the 1950s television series *The Adventures of Fu Manchu*) also has him threaten America with a deadly plague.[30]

Drawing an uncomplicated line from Rohmer to conspiracy theories over a Wuhan lab leak in 2019 would be a mistake, but they both drink deep from the same well. Despite the cosmetic point that official languages around race are supposed to have shifted, it is difficult to interpret the Metropolitan police's designation of victims of racist violence as 'oriental' as somehow discordant or out of step with the events of 2020. When Edward Said's *Orientalism* was published in 1978, he described a long tradition of looking at the global east from the global west, with an exoticizing, shaming, imperialistic gaze.[31] During Covid-19, this gaze resulted in significant violence and harm. As the pandemic wore on, however, it was by no means the only way that racialized bodies were subjected to damaging scrutiny and shame.

The lepers of Leicester

When Manchu taunted the protagonist of *The Mystery of Dr Fu Manchu,* Dr Petrie, with his knowledge of the leper colony on Moloka'i, the implication – that he could, himself, effectively induce leprosy – promised both bodily sickness and social death. On 2 July 2020, the UK government announced the trial of a new public health approach to local and regional restrictions, based on numbers of cases and rates of infection. The announcement of the first 'local lockdown' in the city of Leicester followed from the new policy of identifying and policing specific viral 'hotspots'. As the Scientific Pandemic Insights Group on Behaviours – a sub-group of the Scientific Advisory Group for Emergencies (SAGE) – later reflected, this strategy of identification and isolation allowed shame to accrue around distinct and identifiable cities, towns, neighbourhoods and postcodes.[32] Shame here was the by-product of public health policies which drew national attention to specific places, spotlighting the people who lived there as vectors for disease and raising questions over differences in behaviour as causes for higher rates of transmission.

Like Leicester, these 'hotspots' were frequently places with histories of spatial stigma, or concentrations of communities with long experiences of shaming and racialization.[33] In journalistic and social media discourses, particularly around the city of Leicester, leprosy surfaced as a metaphor for the pariah status that residents were made to endure. National news outlets, for example, reported the experience of a woman from West Knighton,

Tracy Jebbett, who felt that she had been branded a 'Leicester leper' after a holiday park in Cornwall closed its gates to holidaymakers from the city and some of its surrounding areas.[34] Inhabitants of the city felt simultaneously abandoned and hyper-visible, a combination with a heightened potential for shame. Ashamed that they were unable to relax restrictions alongside most of the rest of the country on 4 July 2020, they also believed they were being singled out and punished unfairly.[35] In their dissection of the shaming effect of 'local lockdowns', the SAGE sub-group speculated on the long-term effects of designating areas as Covid-19 'hotspots'; referring specifically to areas in Leicester, they suggested that they could potentially 'become known as a place to avoid for fear of contracting COVID-19', setting patterns of avoidance and disinvestment in process which, if economic decline results, can become self-perpetuating: 'an area that people do not want to visit will become an area in which people do not want to live'.[36]

The local lockdown in Leicester drew together a series of pressure points on shame, racialization and pandemic behaviour. Two studies from the COVID and Care Research Group (CCRG) at the London School of Economics engage extensively with stigma, race and place, taking Leicester as a specific case study and analysing testimony from residents.[37] In their nuanced and detailed work, the CCRG identify overlapping layers of potentially shaming discourses on ethnic minorities and Covid-19. Shame, they argue, is coded into public health vocabularies which attempt to present as innocuous or value-neutral:

Moral languages of pollution, hygiene and recklessness have been used to apportion blame to certain groups. Avoidance of stigmatised populations is often articulated through the oblique language of safety and protection, rather than illness or infection. Conversations about safety are used as a proxy for conversations about transmission and epidemiology; where the language of protection takes the place of the language of illness and infection.[38]

In Leicester, media narratives on multi-generational households, overcrowding, labour conditions and religious observance were used as a proxy to lay the blame for viral transmission at the door of racialized communities, misunderstanding and neglecting important needs, complexities and cultural practices.[39] This resulted in an 'acute legacy' of stigma, with the centre of Leicester City acquiring a lasting reputation as the 'hotzone' or 'dangerzone'.[40] The CCRG conclude that people of colour across the UK have faced a double burden of stigma during Covid-19; a transmission stigma connected with high rates of infection among their communities, and an intensification of 'existing experiences of stigma and racism caused by histories of exclusion, discrimination, and colonialism', with particular groups 'blamed for non-compliance with COVID-19 restrictions'.[41] In a phone-in to the radio station LBC on 31 July, for example, the Conservative MP for Calder Valley, Craig Whittaker, blamed increased restrictions in his constituency on 'the BAME communities that are not taking this seriously enough'.[42]

While Whittaker was condemned for his comments (although not by Boris Johnson), he was only saying the quiet part loud; by announcing a last-minute escalation of quarantine measures on the eve of Eid al-Adha, the Muslim religious festival, Matt Hancock was widely interpreted as implying that Muslim communities in particular were not abiding by social distancing guidelines.[43] Examining anti-Muslim racism in the pandemic, Elizabeth Poole and Milly Williamson situate heightened anxieties around Muslim behaviour and religious observance as an example of how racism 'adapts and stretches over new situations', with old tropes of social threat and lack of integration repackaged for the Covid-19 context.[44]

Race and Covid-19 health inequalities

As early as spring 2020, evidence pointed to the uneven number of Covid-19 infections among ethnic minorities in the UK; in addition, members of racialized communities who contracted the virus were consistently found to be at greater risk of serious symptoms, hospitalization and death than white people of similar age and gender.[45] During the early months of the pandemic, shocking racial disparities in the deaths of doctors and other healthcare workers in the UK gave the first indication that mortality rates might also be skewed at a national level. In March and April 2020, 64 per cent of all nurses and 95 per cent of all doctors who died of Covid-19 were ethnic minorities.[46] The reasons behind these findings are multi-layered, intersecting with other complicated causal relationships between health and structural racism. In terms of infection rates, a number of factors can help to explain the evidence. A disproportionately high presence in the healthcare professions among particular groups – such as Black women from African backgrounds or men from Indian backgrounds – probably results in increased rates of occupational exposure.[47] In the case of healthcare workers, individuals from ethnic minority backgrounds reported higher rates of bullying and harassment during the pandemic, and felt less confident and safe in reporting PPE shortages, with the result that they were more likely than white co-workers to be exposed to the virus.[48] Indeed, some nurses and healthcare assistants from ethnic minority backgrounds felt they were being 'targeted' to work on Covid-19 wards.[49]

In the broader community, minoritised groups generally have higher levels of risk as a result of 'inequalities in exposure to the social determinants of health' where the environments and conditions within which individuals live, work, grow and age – such as their place of employment, housing, their access to goods and services, access to healthcare, and food scarcity or security – cause inequalities in chronic conditions. These in turn increase the severity of Covid-19 infection.[50] Within the UK, ethnic minorities are more likely to live in urban areas, where infection has been higher and social distancing more difficult to achieve. They have been less likely to be able to stop working or work from home, disproportionately making up the workforce in service and frontline positions, directly placing them at higher risk, sometimes even in comparison with white co-workers in the same job. Public health edicts around staying at home, moreover, work from a white middle-class imagining of domestic space which ethnic minorities are frequently excluded from.[51] Even non-compliance with public health guidance, where it actually occurs, has to be understood in the context of historic and understandable mistrust of medical and state authority, and the less than proactive approach taken by the UK government to communicate information in diverse cultural and linguistic contexts.[52]

This phenomenon, in which shame was adroitly shifted away from structural factors and placed squarely with racialized communities, was reproduced even more insidiously in the lack of a sincere public reckoning with the relationship between racism and reduced health outcomes. Literatures on minority stress, the psychological and physical burden of racism, and significant and pervasive health inequalities among racialized groups are well evidenced and well established.[53] While heightened hospitalization and mortality rates among ethnic minorities with Covid-19 had genuine public visibility and cut-through, politicians, media outlets and prominent health advisors largely abdicated responsibility for explaining where and how these disparities originated. Despite good, early evidence on why infection, morbidity and mortality rates might be higher among particular communities, there was a comprehensive political failure to engage publicly with structural racism as a causative factor for health inequalities in Covid-19. The publication of the Sewell Report (the findings of the Commission on Race and Ethnic Disparities) in March 2021, a document which has been described by the Runnymede Trust as 'frankly disturbing' in its suggestion that 'institutional racism does not exist', represented the culmination of a long refusal on the part of conservative politicians to acknowledge that racism in the UK exceeds the isolated behaviour of individual bad actors.[54] In the deliberate fixation on individual responsibility and behaviour in public health, media and political rhetoric (see Chapters 1 and 5 of this volume), racist anxieties about disease transmission, culturally contingent living arrangements and the misuse of public and private space were allowed to fill a discursive gap between undeniable facts and figures (in the form of publicly visible epidemiological data on inequalities in Covid outcomes) and the uncomfortable and jarring context required to make them explicable. As Vanessa Apea and Yize Wan point out in their response to the Sewell Report, the Covid-19 pandemic has in fact been a peerless illustration of the existence of structural racism, with the accompanying denial acting as an important component of its perpetuation.[55]

Although sometimes complicated, structural narratives on Covid-19, systemic racism and health inequality are by no means impossible to publicly communicate. In terms of public health evidence, homogenizing categories such as BAME have limited explanatory value. Granular, intersectional work on how members of particular groups are subject to structural racism in specific places and contexts is necessary to fully illuminate the myriad pathways to poorer health outcomes, both in Covid-19 and in general. Data on outcome disparities within these loose categories, however, could have been accompanied by a broad-strokes, unequivocal analysis of the entrenched structures of exclusion and oppression which frame the health and illness experiences of racialized people in the UK.

In simplistic and general terms, racism impacts health in three ways. It directly erodes physical and mental health through long processes of attrition, particularly through the stress and shame of racialization, discrimination and overt prejudice.[56] This includes the fear or experience of racist violence, over-policing, public scrutiny and stigmatizing medical and public health interventions. Structural racism also frequently results in poor living and working conditions, material poverty and deprivation, and reduced educational opportunities. These social and economic determinants of health impose an additional physical, psychological and relational burden, deepening and complicating other experiences of ill-health.[57] In both instances, a cyclical relationship between physical and mental comorbidities, and between health and environment, can decrease health-seeking behaviour; it can also contribute to premature ageing, or 'weathering', through the sustained application of psychosocial, physical and chemical stressors.[58] Structural racism further affects how and whether racialized people engage with healthcare services and public health messaging, how they are treated in clinical encounters, and which kinds of health conditions are prioritized within NHS planning and resource allocation.[59]

Particularly in the context of a government committed to denying the structural nature of racism, its indisputable inscription on the minds and bodies of British citizens is a profoundly shaming and exposing legacy. As with inequalities in infection rates, this deliberate omission deflected shame from institutions, ideologies and structures, allowing it to attach to individual factors and decisions. This can be read as a cynical and complicit exercise in saving face. Presented with decontextualized data on disparities in morbidity and mortality, different communities were left to speculate on what might explain them. Some placed in the 'BAME' category attributed their 'clinical vulnerability' to genetic predispositions, or to long-standing chronic diseases caused by 'lifestyle and diet'.[60] This internalization of deflected shame over Covid-19 entrenches and deepens the cyclical burden of structural racism and health inequality, afflicting populations which have already been rendered shame-prone by long experiences of social shaming.

Coughing while Asian

'Coughing while Asian' brought acute bodily shame over the potential transmission of disease into close proximity with deeper structures of racialized shaming. Tow and Arboleda's film actively set out to satirize and subvert these shame dynamics; T-shirts bearing the legend 'Lestah Lepers', featuring the city's fox mascot in a gas mask, can be found for sale online. These attempts at levity, however, were tangled up with real suffering and stress. The Mass Observation respondent who wrote that she felt 'very Asian in public' recounted that she began online therapy after these experiences, joining a growing population of service users across the global West seeking urgent psychological support for race-based trauma during the pandemic.[61] Direct experiences of overt racism and violence are significant life events, with serious consequences for emotional, physiological and relational health. They cast a long shadow, introducing damaging patterns of fear and shame which can be difficult to break out of. For members of racialized groups routinely (or acutely) subject to violence and abuse, anticipated experiences and the experiences of others can be a persistent source of anxiety and collective pain.[62] Far from trivial, social slights, microaggressions, hypervisibility and exaggerated physical avoidance also take a cumulative toll. The 'new' body language of social distancing reproduces and reformulates the 'old' body language of stigma and suspicion, with different consequences for communities with long experiences of being avoided or snubbed by white people.[63] Although there are rapidly emerging literatures on anti-Asian racism, health inequalities and Covid-19, our analysis suggests an ongoing need to engage with literatures on shame. Shame is an under-recognized and under-explored component of acute and structural racism, and chronic shame is an important theoretical device in understanding how processes of exclusion and stigmatization actively translate into poor health.[64]

Attempts to shame people of East and Southeast Asian backgrounds with culpability for the transmission and origins of Covid-19 tapped into older and deeper structures of racialized shaming, following cultural scripts which have been well-established for over a century. Likewise, with a political, media and scientific establishment largely unprepared to acknowledge structural racism and its effects on health, shaming narratives on individual responsibility, behaviour and choice were allowed to fill the information gap accompanying 'BAME' mortality and morbidity data. The most comprehensive failure, a recent study of ethnic disparities in Covid-19 suggests, is our systemic cultural and political refusal to confront shameful histories: 'Many high income countries with legacies of slavery, imperialism and colonialism have a moral duty to reckon with the past. We know the problems, and the solutions are mostly in front of us.'[65] Predictably, attempts to do precisely that, in the form of the Black Lives Matter protests prompted by the murder of George Floyd on 25 May 2020 – as well as the police taking no further action in the case of Belly Mujinga, a transport worker who died in April after alleging that a man who claimed to have Covid had spat on her in her place of work – were subject to extensive criticism and censure for spreading the virus, including by Matt Hancock. Critics of Black Lives Matter deliberately sidestepped the question of precisely what kinds of survival were at stake in the 'twin pandemics' of Covid-19 and racism.[66]

In disowning that moral duty, the UK government knowingly increased the burden of shame on ethnic minorities, rendering them publicly culpable both for their own bodies and behaviour, and for a civic imagining of collective health which had always excluded and neglected them. As the following chapter explores, racialized bodies were not alone in subjection to alienating and intrusive systems of policing, surveillance and shame, with neoliberal languages of individual responsibility and choice eliding and obscuring important social, economic and relational determinants of health. Nor were they the only context in which significant evidence on shame in public health was comprehensively ignored, or where long histories of medical and cultural humiliation and disgust culminated in poorer outcomes for chronically shamed populations.

Notes

1. Tow-Arboleda Films, 'Coughing while Asian Corona Virus', 3 February 2021. Video and accompanying text. https://www.youtube.com/watch?v=HZq7fwUywR4.

2. Lauren Aratini, '"Coughing while Asian": Living in Fear as Racism Feeds off Coronavirus Panic', *The Guardian*, 24 March 2020, 22.00 GMT. https://www.theguardian.com/world/2020/mar/24/coronavirus-us-asian-americans-racism.

3. David A. Harris, 'Driving While Black: Racial Profiling on Our Nation's Motorways', *American Civil Liberties Union Special Report*, June 1999. https://www.aclu.org/report/driving-while-black-racial-profiling-our-nations-highways; Leonore F. Carpenter and R. Barrett Marshall, 'Walking while Trans: Profiling of Transgender Women by Law Enforcement, and the Problem of Proof', *William & Mary Journal of Women and the Law* vol. 24:1 (2017), 5–38.

4. Aratini, 'Coughing while Asian'.

5. Karen Dunn, 'Conservative Leader's "bat soup" Comments Not a Code of Conduct Breach', *Sussex Express*, 25 January 2021. https://www.sussexexpress.co.uk/news/politics/conservative-leaders-bat-soup-comments-not-a-code-of-conduct-breach-3111501.

6. Matthew Sparke and Owain David Williams, 'Neoliberal Disease: COVID-19, Co-Pathogenesis and Global Health Insecurities', *Environment and Planning A: Economy and Space* vol. 54:1 (February 2022), 15–32, 16. https://doi.org/10.1177/0308518X211048905.

7. Hansard HC Deb 13 October 2020, vol. 682, col. 114. https://hansard.parliament.uk/commons/2020-10-13/debates/858E78B5-1049-4480-A1A7-5362FC12F47E/ChineseAndEastAsianCommunitiesRacismDuringCovid-19.

8. Mass Observation Archive (University of Sussex): Replies to Spring 2020 Directive [R7180].

9. Hansard HC Deb 13 October 2020, vol 682, col 114.

10. Nini Fang and Shan-Jan Sarah Liu, 'Critical Conversations: Being Yellow Women in the Time of COVID-19', *International Feminist Journal of Politics* vol. 23:2 (2021), 333–40. https://doi.org/10.1080/14616742.2021.1894969.

11. Hannah Farrimond, 'Stigma Mutation: Tracking Lineage, Variation and Strength in Emerging COVID-19 Stigma', *Sociological Research Online* (August 2021), 1–18. https://doi.org/10.1177/13607804211031580.

12. Ditch the Label, 'Uncovered: Online Hate Speech in the Covid Era', November 2021. https://www.ditchthelabel.org/research-papers/hate-speech-report-2021/.

13. Melissa Harris-Perry, *Sister Citizen: Shame, Stereotypes and Black Women in America* (New Haven and London: Yale University Press, 2011).

14. Aness Kim Webster, 'Making Sense of Shame in Response to Racism', *Canadian Journal of Philosophy,* 51:7 (2021), 535–50, 543.

15. Webster, 'Making Sense of Shame in Response to Racism', 547.

16. Billie Thomson, 'Chinese Woman Eats Bat in Restaurant Despite Coronavirus Link', *MailOnline*, 23 January 2020. https://www.dailymail.co.uk/news/article-7920573/Revolting-footage-shows-Chinese-woman-eating-bat-scientists-link-coronavirus-animal.html.

17. James Palmer, 'Don't Blame Bat Soup for the Coronavirus', *Foreign Policy*, 27 January 2020. https://foreignpolicy.com/2020/01/27/coronavirus-covid19-dont-blame-bat-soup-for-the-virus/.

18. Roger Luckhurst, 'The Chinese Virus', *Critical Quarterly* vol. 62:4 (December 2020), 54–62, 55. https://doi.org/10.1111/criq.12582.

19. Stephen L. Muzzatti, 'Bits of Falling Sky and Global Pandemics: Moral Panic and Severe Acute Respiratory Syndrome (SARS)', *Illness, Crisis & Loss* vol. 13:2 (April 2005), 117–28. https://doi.org/10.1177/105413730501300203; Katherine A. Mason, 'H1N1 Is Not a Chinese Virus: The Racialization of People and Viruses in Post-SARS China', *Studies in Comparative International Development* vol. 50:4 (2015), 500–18. https://doi.org/10.1007/s12116-015-9198-y.

20. Des Fitzgerald, 'Normal Island: COVID-19, Border Control, and Viral Nationalism in UK Public Health Discourse', *Sociological Research Online* (November 2021). https://doi.org/10.1177/13607804211049464.

21. Hansard HC Deb 13 October 2020, vol 682, col 113.

22. Daniel Renshaw, 'Prejudice and Paranoia: A Comparative Study of Antisemitism and Sinophobia in Turn-of-the-century Britain', *Patterns of Prejudice* vol. 50:1 (2016), 38–60, 17, 21. https://doi.org/10.1080/0031322X.2015.1127646.

23. Luckhurst, 'The Chinese Virus'.

24. Anne Witchard, *England's Yellow Peril: Sinophobia and the Great War* (London: Penguin, 2014), 28–9.

25. Jacques Schnier, 'Morphology of a Symbol: The Octopus', *American Imago* vol. 13:1 (1956), 3–31.

26. Renshaw, 'Prejudice and Paranoia', 23.

27. Luckhurst, 'The Chinese Virus', 60.

28. Sax Rohmer, *The Mystery of Dr. Fu-Manchu* (1913), https://www.gutenberg.org/files/173/173-h/173-h.htm, Chapter XIII.

29. R. D. K. Herman, 'Out of Sight, Out of Mind, Out of Power: Leprosy, Race, and Colonization in Hawai'i', *Hulili: Multidisciplinary Research on Hawaiian Well-Being* vol. 6 (2010), 265–96, 275; Renisa Mawani, "'The Island of the Unclean": Race, Colonialism and "Chinese Leprosy" in British Columbia, 1891–1924', *Law, Social Justice & Global Development Journal* vol. 1 (2003). https://warwick.ac.uk/fac/soc/law/elj/lgd/2003_1/mawani/.

30. Luckhurst, 'The Chinese Virus', 61.

31. Edward W. Said, *Orientalism* (New York: Pantheon Books, 1978).

32. Scientific Pandemic Insights Group on Behaviours, 'SPI-B: Health status Certification in Relation to COVID-19, Behavioural and Social Considerations', 9 December 2020, 13. https://www.gov.uk/government/publications/spi-b-health-status-certification-in-relation-to-covid-19-behavioural-and-social-considerations-9-december-2020.

33. Emma Halliday et al., 'The Elephant in The Room? Why Spatial Stigma Does Not Receive the Public Health Attention It Deserves', *Journal of Public Health* vol. 42:1 (2020), 38–43. https://doi.org/10.1093/pubmed/fdy214.

34. Coronavirus: 'I Felt Like I Was being Penalised', *BBC News*, 30 June 2020. https://www.bbc.co.uk/news/uk-england-cornwall-53237240.

35. Laura Bear et al., 'A Right to Care: The Social Foundations of Recovery from Covid-19', *Covid and Care Research Group*, 22 October 2020, 94. https://www.lse.ac.uk/anthropology/assets/documents/research/Covid-and-Care/ARighttoCare-CovidandCare-Final-2310.pdf.

36. Scientific Pandemic Insights Group on Behaviours, 'SPI-B', 6.

37. Bear et al., 'A Right to Care'; Laura Bear et al., 'Social Infrastructures for the post-Covid recovery in the UK', Covid and Care Research Group, 12 July 2021. http://eprints.lse.ac.uk/111011/4/SocialInfrastructures_ReportFinal_180122.pdf.

38. Bear et al., 'A Right to Care', 85.

39. Bear et al., 'A Right to Care', 89, 95.

40. Bear et al., 'Social Infrastructures for the post-Covid recovery in the UK', 58.

41. Bear et al., 'Social Infrastructures for the Post-Covid recovery in the UK', 54.

42. Adrian Sherling, 'Muslim and BAME Communities Not Taking Coronavirus Pandemic Seriously', *Tory MP says*', LBC, 31 July 2020, 08:33. https://www.lbc.co.uk/radio/presenters/ian-payne/muslim-bame-communities-coronavirus-pandemic/.

43. Josh Halliday and Guy Kilty, 'Hancock Added to Anti-Muslim Hate with Distancing Claims, Says Government Adviser', *The Guardian*, 26 October 2020, 11.18 GMT. https://www.theguardian.com/uk-news/2020/oct/26/hancock-added-to-anti-muslim-hate-with-distancing-claims-says-government-adviser.

44. Elizabeth Poole and Milly Williamson, 'How Racist Narratives about Muslims in the British Press Were Reconfigured during the Initial Peak of COVID-19', *LSE British Politics and Policy*, 7 September 2021. https://blogs.lse.ac.uk/politicsandpolicy/press-reporting-muslims-covid19/.

45. Office for National Statistics, 'Coronavirus (COVID-19) Related Deaths by Ethnic Group, England and Wales: 2 March 2020 to 10 April 2020', 7 May 2020. https://www.ons.gov.uk/peoplepopulationandcommunity/birthsdeathsandmarriages/deaths/articles/coronavirusrelateddeathsbyethnicgroupenglandandwales/2march2020to10april2020.

46. British Medical Association, 'COVID-19: The Risk to BAME Doctors', 24 August 2021. https://www.bma.org.uk/advice-and-support/covid-19/your-health/covid-19-the-risk-to-bame-doctors.

47. Lucinda Platt and Ross Warwick, 'Are Some Ethnic Groups More Vulnerable to COVID-19 Than Others?', *The Institute for Fiscal Studies*, May 2020, 3. https://ifs.org.uk/inequality/wp-content/uploads/2020/04/Are-some-ethnic-groups-more-vulnerable-to-COVID-19-than-others-IFS-Briefing-Note.pdf.

48. British Medical Association, 'COVID-19: The Risk to BAME Doctors'.

49. Megan Ford, 'Exclusive: BME Nurses "feel targeted" to Work on Covid-19 Wards', *Nursing Times*, 17 April 2020. https://www.nursingtimes.net/news/coronavirus/exclusive-bme-nurses-feel-targeted-to-work-on-covid-19-wards-17-04-2020/.

50. Clare Bambra et al., 'The COVID-19 Pandemic and Health Inequalities', *Journal of Epidemiology and Community Health* vol. 74:11 (2020), 964–8, 965. https://doi.org/10.1136/jech-2020-214401.

51. Peter Phiri et al., 'COVID-19 and Black, Asian, and Minority Ethnic Communities: A Complex Relationship without Just Cause', *JMIR Public Health Surveillance* vol. 7:2 (2021), 2, 3. https://doi.org/10.2196/22581.

52. Bear et al., 'A Right to Care', 87.

53. Mohammad S. Razai et al., 'Mitigating Ethnic Disparities in Covid-19 and beyond', *British Medical Journal* 372, 15 January 2021. https://doi.org/10.1136/bmj.m4921.

54. Commission on Race and Ethnic Disparities, 'The Report of the Commission on Race and Ethnic Disparities', 31 March 2021. https://assets.publishing.service.gov.uk/government/uploads/system/uploads/attachment_data/file/974507/20210331_-_CRED_Report_-_FINAL_-_Web_Accessible.pdf; Harriet Whitehead, 'Charities Criticise "frankly disturbing" Sewell Race Report', *Civil Society*, 6 April 2021. https://www.civilsociety.co.uk/news/charities-hit-back-at-frankly-disturbing-sewell-race-report.html.

55. Vanessa Apea and Yize Wan, 'Yes, There Is Structural Racism in the UK – COVID-19 Outcomes Prove It', *The Conversation*, 6 April 2021, 7.27pm BST. https://theconversation.com/yes-there-is-structural-racism-in-the-uk-covid-19-outcomes-prove-it-158337.

56. Yin Paradies et al., 'Racism as a Determinant of Health: A Systematic Review and Meta-Analysis', *PLOS ONE* vol. 10:9 (2015). https://doi.org/10.1371/journal.pone.0138511.

57. Luna Dolezal and Barry Lyons, 'Health-related Shame: An Affective Determinant of Health?', *Medical Humanities* vol. 43:4 (2017), 257–63. https://doi.org/10.1136/medhum-2017-011186.

58. Razai et al., 'Mitigating Ethnic Disparities in Covid-19 and Beyond'; A.T. Geronimus, 'The Weathering Hypothesis and the Health of African-American Women and Infants: Evidence and Speculations', *Ethnicity and Disease* vol. 2:3 (1992), 207–21.

59. Phiri et al., 'COVID-19 and Black, Asian, and Minority Ethnic Communities', 2.

60. Bear et al., 'A Right to Care', 87.

61. Mass Observation Archive: Replies to Spring 2020 Directive [R7180]; Stacey Diane A. Litam, '"Take your Kung-Flu back to Wuhan": Counseling Asians, Asian Americans, and pacific Islanders with Race-based Trauma Related to COVID-19', *The Professional Counselor* vol. 10:2 (2020), 144–56. https://doi.org/10.15241/sdal.10.2.144.

62. David R Williams et al., 'Racism and Health: Evidence and Needed Research', *Annual Review of Public Health* vol. 40 (2019), 105–25. https://doi.org/10.1146/annurev-publhealth-040218-043750.

63. Luna Dolezal and Gemma Lucas, 'Differential Experiences of Social Distancing: Considering Alienated Embodied Communication and Racism', *Puncta: Journal of Critical Phenomenology* vol 5:1 (2022), 97–105.

64. Harris-Perry, *Sister Citizen;* Dolezal and Lyons, 'Health-Related Shame: An Affective Determinant of Health?', 260.

65. Razai et al., 'Mitigating Ethnic Disparities in Covid-19 and Beyond', 4.

66. Adam Tooze, *Shutdown: How Covid Shook the World's Economy* (London: Allen Lane, 2021), 36; Craig A. Harper and Darren Rhode, 'Ideological Responses to the Breaking of COVID-19 Social Distancing Recommendations', *Group Processes and Intergroup Relations* (preprint). https://doi.org/10.31234/osf.io/dkqj6; 'Anti-Racism Protests Undoubtedly Increase Risk of Coronavirus Spread -UK Health Minister', *Reuters*, 7 June 2020. https://www.reuters.com/article/health-coronavirus-britain-protests-idUSL8N2DK03F; Sari Altschuler and Priscilla Wald, 'COVID-19 and the Language of Racism', *Signs: Feminists Theorize COVID-19*, http://signsjournal.org/covid/altschuler-and-wald/; Lucy Campbell, 'Belly Mujinga: Family Still Seeking Justice One Year after Covid Death', *The Guardian*, Mon 5 April 2021. 16.10 BST. https://www.theguardian.com/world/2021/apr/05/belly-mujinga-family-still-seeking-justice-one-year-after-covid-death.

CHAPTER 4
I WAS TOO FAT: BORIS JOHNSON AND THE FAT PANIC

27 March 2020. Boris Johnson is in self-isolation after testing positive for Covid-19. Rumours circulate that he is seriously ill, but the official message from Number 10 Downing Street remains that his symptoms are mild. What follows is a national 'emotional rollercoaster'.[1] At first, the public are reassured that all is well. Johnson himself appears on video eight days into his self-isolation. 'Although I'm feeling better', he confides, 'alas I still have … a minor symptom … I still have a temperature'.[2] The press are assured that Johnson is likely to emerge from isolation the following day. Behind the scenes, however, a very different picture is forming. St Thomas' hospital has already begun preparations to admit him, as it seems increasingly likely Johnson will need oxygen support. The prime minister is very unwell and deteriorating rapidly.

Over the weekend of the 4th and 5th of April, the government continued to insist that Johnson was only mildly ill, with the health secretary Matt Hancock claiming on Sunday that Johnson was still 'working away' with his 'hand on the tiller'.[3] Later that day, Johnson was admitted to hospital and Number 10 didn't deny that he was immediately given oxygen.[4] Despite the obvious seriousness of the prime minister's condition, there was a continued insistence that Johnson was fine. For example, the foreign secretary Dominic Raab stated at the 5pm daily press briefing for Monday the 6th of April that Johnson was 'admitted to hospital for tests as a precaution only' and that 'he remains in charge of the government'.[5]

For journalists and the public, it remained unclear to what extent the government was conspiring to cover up the seriousness of Johnson's illness. 'Things took an almost Soviet turn', as one journalist put it, as the government kept insisting on the farce that Johnson was fine, when he so clearly wasn't. Indeed, on Monday a few hours after Raab's declaration that Johnson was still 'in charge', Johnson was transferred to St Thomas's intensive care unit, where beds were generally reserved for patients needing to be put on ventilators. Raab later claimed that he had no idea about the sudden worsening of Johnson's condition and hadn't spoken to Johnson since Saturday.

Johnson remained in the intensive care unit for three nights; although he received oxygen support, he was never put on mechanical ventilation. Johnson's health began to improve, and he was eventually discharged after seven nights in hospital, returning to Chequers, his official country residence, on Sunday the 12th of April. Although his father, Stanley, claimed that Boris 'almost took one for the Team',[6] the prime minister went on to make a full recovery and his personal experience of contracting Covid-19 and falling seriously ill went on to shape government policy.

On 27 July 2020, just over three months later, the UK government launched the 'Better Health' campaign, a public health initiative marketed explicitly as related to Boris Johnson's experience of having Covid-19. To coincide with the launch of this campaign, Number 10 released a social media video of Johnson walking his dog Dilyn in the park and speaking candidly about his own experience: 'When I went into ICU, when I was really ill, I was way overweight.' The inspirational music builds as Johnson eventually declares, 'you know, I was too fat'.[7] Johnson elaborated this message during his speech at the virtual Conservative Party conference in October: 'The reason I had such a nasty experience with the disease is that although I was superficially in the pink of health when I caught it, I had a very common underlying condition.' After a three second pause, he drives it home with a smirk: 'My friends, I was too fat.'[8]

At this stage, the links between obesity and mortality rates from Covid-19 had been emphasized by the government for months, with a Public Health England Report released on 25 July 2020, just days before the launch of the Tackling Obesity strategy. This report outlined evidence that the risk of hospitalization, intensive care admission and death from Covid-19 was greater for those who were severely overweight, with the risk growing substantially as BMI increased.[9] Statistics showed that while 7.9 per cent of critically ill Covid-19 patients in intensive care in the UK had been classified as morbidly obese (where one is at least 100 pounds over 'ideal' body weight), the number in the general population was only 2.9 per cent.[10] The reasons for this were both physiological and psycho-social, as Public Health England summarized:

Excess fat can affect the respiratory system and is likely to affect inflammatory and immune function. This can impact people's response to infection and increase vulnerability to severe symptoms of

COVID-19. Obese people may be less likely to access healthcare and support, and it is also thought that COVID-19 affects other diseases associated with obesity.[11]

The correlation between being overweight and the risk of ending up in an NHS hospital because of Covid-19 was undeniable. In Number 10's social media video, the message from the prime minister on this point is explicit. As the music swells, Johnson outlines some of the personal benefits to weight loss and exercise: 'you feel much better … you feel more full of energy', finally adding offhandedly, and almost apologetically: 'And you know, the other thing, obviously is that if you can get your weight down a bit, and then protect your health, you'll also be protecting the NHS.'[12]

In this chapter, we examine how the government's response to excess weight and obesity during Covid-19 followed the discourse espoused by the prime minister after his own experience of contracting Covid-19, recovering and losing weight. The official public health policy was underscored by an emphasis on the 'costs' of obesity, particularly to the NHS, and an insistence that individuals' 'choices' could offer a solution. This explicit public health strategy positioned individuals living with excess weight as recipients of shame, blame and moral outrage, not only for their own failures to lose weight but also for putting undue strain on the NHS and its resources. Fuelled by a Covid-19 related 'fat panic',[13] we argue, fat shaming became an implicit, and sometimes explicit, public health strategy during 2020. This approach seemed to ignore both the context within which anti-obesity policies were developed and the public health evidence demonstrating that obesity and excess weight are deeply correlated with complex social issues such as food insecurity, poverty, inequality and social deprivation, all of which have been largely exacerbated during Covid-19 as a result of lockdowns and other restrictions.

Post-war approaches to obesity

In the UK, post-war approaches to obesity were conditioned by a series of contexts: experiences and memories of rationing and austerity; pre-existing welfarist concerns around diet, hunger and malnutrition; and the creation of the NHS.[14] Under rationing, excess weight acted as a potential signifier of over-consumption of – and therefore unfair access to – food, isolating specific kinds of bodies from the kinship of shared struggle.[15] As weight gain became more common during 1950s affluence, the causes and consequences of obesity were largely individualized; literatures on diet proliferated, but discussions of the 'cost' revolved mostly around personal inability to participate in a particular kind of carefree and attractive sociality.

If not exactly representing a critique of affluence, this lens on obesity sought to draw out the unintended consequences of choice; with consumption no longer regulated by the state, individuals were 'free' to pursue diets which could be inimical to individual and family health. According to Martha Kirby, the tenor of debate shifted decisively in the years following the publication of the 'Build and Blood Pressure Study' by the Metropolitan Life Insurance Company in 1959.[16] In relating obesity to heart disease, the problem was re-framed in terms of extra-individual cost, with the NHS and the economy as public victims of private choices.

Relating private choices to public costs created ample room for shame and shaming. Kirby cites the 1967 public information film *A Cruel Kindness*, issued by the British Medical Association and the British Life Assurance Trust for Health Education. The film discusses one character as a 'fat, breathless woman' who makes 'matters worse by stuffing her family with a stodgy meal'.[17] In her work on quantification, obesity and the cultural history of the NHS, Roberta Bivins quotes the Greenwich Medical Officer for Health, J. Kerr Brown, as follows: 'the aim of health education is to achieve a climate of opinion where indulgence in anti-health activities is viewed with the same distaste as infrequent bathing, spitting, etc.'.[18] In short, the aim of public health communication is to use shame and disgust as affective drivers to 'motivate' individuals to avoid certain lifestyle choices, like excessive 'indulgence', which could lead to health complications like excess weight or heart disease.

Simultaneously, counter-narratives emerged which attempted to sensitize policymakers to the political, economic, environmental and social contexts of excess weight, and which laid the foundations for the structural approach to obesity in which our critique is situated. Unfortunately, as the historian Jane Hand explores, interventions on health inequalities (such as the Black Report in 1980) were limited in their influence on policy, as subsequent governments framed disparities, including around health, as 'not inherently structural but rather the outcome of personal choice, which could therefore be overcome by individual commitment, skill, and motivation'.[19] This is not a side-product of neoliberal politics but a governing logic. A partial re-investment in understanding and addressing complex determinants of health under New Labour (1997–2010) had not been able to – and was not necessarily intended to – sufficiently trouble an ingrained cultural conflation of excess weight with greed or lack of self-restraint, although it may have allowed for a more nuanced media discussion of obesity than has subsequently been the case. Research into the framing of the obesity 'problem' in UK newspapers between 2008 and 2017 has demonstrated that references to the responsibilities of government or the food industry have decreased over time.[20]

Threaded throughout the question of responsibility (or blame) for obesity, the problem of cost to the NHS has been used as a central basis for shaming fat bodies. Bivins locates the beginnings of this process in debates about the high cost of 'slimming drugs' in the late 1970s, resurfacing in perennial anxieties about resource scarcity, system failure, and the NHS as 'under threat' from citizens' unnecessary and irresponsible health choices. Journalistic expositions on obesity, through the 1990s, 2000s and 2010s, were frequently accompanied by quantifications of the financial costs.[21] In their examination of changing media scripts on obesity, Baker et al. reproduce a relatively representative passage from *The Daily Telegraph* in 2014: 'the obese are gobbling up limited NHS services and costing taxpayers more than 55 million a year'.[22] This imposed a further dimension to weight shame, with the harms of obesity redistributed to 'good' citizens who had to shoulder the burden of those who, unlike themselves, were unwilling to regulate their appetites and manage their health. The 2020 Tackling Obesity initiative reconfigured this shaming and dehumanizing narrative, but the building blocks are the same: the NHS as under threat, and people with excess weight as complicit, selfish and worthy of shame.[23]

Neoliberalism and fat shaming

The assumptions guiding anti-obesity public health strategies since the 1980s in the UK have been broadly underpinned and guided by a neoliberal ideological framework, a framework that has increasingly infiltrated healthcare services in many Western countries where reforms are focused on privatization resulting in the dismantling and weakening of nationally funded healthcare systems.[24] Throughout the late 1980s and the 1990s, healthcare reform followed neoliberal principles of providing greater competition and consumer power for patients, which led to the significant privatization of NHS services.[25] These market reforms have, David Sturgeon argues, 'transformed the NHS from a single national healthcare provider to a fragmented conglomeration of competing services delivering healthcare under the umbrella of the NHS brand'.[26] Not only has a neoliberal framework dominated the way that publicly funded healthcare is delivered and organized, it has also reshaped the way we generally consider the achievement of 'health' and 'wellbeing' to come about. Through neoliberal logics, 'health' and 'wellbeing' have become pursuits and achievements of individuals, where the responsibility for good health is placed firmly on an individual's ability to regulate, manage and invest in their own lifestyle, body and health-related activities.[27] This individualization of responsibility means that poor health and other social ills, like poverty and unemployment, are often seen as an individual shortcoming and the result of poor lifestyle choices.[28]

The neoliberal emphasis on individual self-management, self-control and self-actualization has led to, as Hannele Harjunen argues, body size and the economy becoming 'closely intertwined with each other'.[29] The good neoliberal citizen has a particular body type: they are attractive, affluent, stylish, in good shape and, of course, slender. A very visible marker of what is commonly thought of as a 'bad' or 'failed' neoliberal citizen is being overweight or obese, where, as Tanisha Spratt notes, 'their excess weight [is] seen as an external marker and/or signifier of their presumed lack of self-control and self-discipline when it comes to food intake and exercise'.[30] Portrayed as lazy, greedy and irresponsible in the dominant cultural imaginary, individuals living with excess weight are routinely positioned in a way that results in routine experiences of shame and shaming.

In her book *Fat Shame*, Amy Farrell argues that fat stigma in the present day is centrally related to 'anxieties over consumer excess', where the 'connotations of fatness and the fat person' are 'lazy, gluttonous, greedy, immoral, uncontrolled, stupid, ugly and lacking in will power'.[31] In short, the dominant assumption is that individuals become overweight because they cannot control and regulate themselves appropriately within a free market environment – they simply make poor choices regarding food intake and exercise. Because of this assumption, 'the fat body is constructed as a kind of "anti-neoliberal" body that is unproductive, ineffective and unprofitable'.[32] In this way, body size has become an immediate and 'crucial marker of social status', and a means through which to measure 'one's suitability for the privileges and power of full citizenship' in the dominant economic and social order.[33] Evidence shows that people who live with excess weight or obesity can have more difficulty achieving employment, promotion and acceptance into university when compared to people who are considered to be slender.[34]

As a result, in our dominant cultural order, being obese or overweight immediately marks an individual as 'inferior', somehow 'less than' optimal.

They are a citizen who has failed to live up to societal expectations, who is not only failing themselves but also failing others and society. As *The Daily Telegraph* quote above demonstrates, these individuals are often blamed for putting strain on public health systems, 'gobbling up limited NHS services', while also putting a large strain on the public purse, 'costing taxpayers more than 55 million a year'. Individuals who are overweight or obese are portrayed as selfishly hogging resources that could benefit others. These 'others' are seen as more deserving, as they are not to blame for their illnesses or conditions. As Harjunen notes:

> The assumed 'choice' to be fat (out of moral incompetence) is then used to justify the discrimination and shaming of fat people … the stigmatisation of fatness [is] more widespread, public and socially acceptable. Public monitoring, surveillance and outright 'policing' of (fat) bodies by the media, health professionals and even the general public is pervasive.[35]

Fat shaming, Spratt writes, 'is a practice where people living with overweight or obesity are purposefully stigmatized and made to feel ashamed because of their body size'.[36] In the UK, people living with overweight and obesity routinely experience fat shaming; it is used as a 'tool', Spratt notes, to both communicate the risks associated with obesity and also to motivate people to lose weight.[37] People living with excess weight or obesity are both *shamed* and *blamed*. They are believed to have directly caused their body size, along with any related health conditions, through poor lifestyle choices.[38] This moral deficit, worthy of blame, is presumed to be caused by an individual's intrinsically flawed character, which signals an ontological deficit that is worthy of shame. Hence, contemporary fat shaming is intrinsically bound up with neoliberal logics which claim that each individual is responsible for their own self-making, their own success and, as a result, their position in the social order. Any failure or lack of success is shamefully *one's own fault*.

The Tackling Obesity campaign

Not surprisingly, the logics of fat shaming and neoliberalism dominated the UK government's response to obesity during the Covid-19 pandemic.[39] As evidence emerged from the UK and France that a disproportionate number of patients admitted to intensive care units with Covid-19 were obese,[40] a 'fat panic' took hold in the UK's public health agenda. Within six months of the start of the pandemic, an explicit campaign to reduce obesity levels in the UK, the Tackling Obesity strategy, was launched.[41] The campaign focused on 'tackling obesity', with the overt aims to 'improve the health of the nation', 'offer greater protection against the impact of COVID-19' and 'protect the NHS from being overwhelmed' in the event of a second wave, or subsequent waves, of the virus.[42]

This campaign was explicitly linked to Boris Johnson's own experience of contracting Covid-19 and being 'too fat'.[43] In the social media video released by Number 10 to coincide with the launch of the campaign, Johnson confesses, 'I've always wanted to lose weight for ages and ages … and like … many people, I struggle with my weight'.[44] Johnson goes on to describe how, after recovering from his illness, he started jogging in the morning and lost weight as a result of changes to his routine and lifestyle.[45] Modelling Johnson's own approach to weight loss following his illness, the UK's new obesity strategy targets change and choice on an individual level, promoting healthy eating, physical activity and weight loss.

Endorsing the Tackling Obesity campaign is a remarkable change of tack for a prime minister well known for his outspoken views regarding the right to unfettered food choices and his opposition to 'nanny state' government interventions that promote healthy eating. In 2006, he is reported as commenting the following on Jamie Oliver's well-known campaign for healthy school meals: 'If I was in charge I would get rid of Jamie Oliver and tell people to eat what they like … I say let people eat what they like. Why shouldn't they push pies through [school] railings … this pressure to bring in healthy food is too much.'[46] In stark contrast to his previous position, now that Johnson *is* in charge, he has sanctioned and supported a national health campaign with a central goal of encouraging healthier food choices made by individuals.

This approach of targeting change and choice on an individual level is not new. In fact, the Tackling Obesity campaign is a further iteration of anti-obesity public health policies that have been in place in the UK for over a decade, starting with the Change4Life anti-obesity campaign, launched in 2009, where individuals were encouraged to make 'smart swaps' to cut sugar and fat from their diets through simple substitutions.[47] The policy paper outlining the details of Tackling Obesity states that it aims to 'empower people to make the healthier choices they want to make'.[48] The 'Better Health' campaign's tagline is the injunction 'Let's do this!' suggesting individual actions to achieve a collective goal. These injunctions to individual-level change regarding exercise and food choices are coupled with measures that address some societal-level issues, such as ensuring calorie counts are included on some restaurant menus, limiting the advertisement and promotion of unhealthy food in shops and on television, and expanding weight management services. However, it should be noted that even these supposedly 'societal-level' changes come down to individual choices regarding which foods to consume, along with which health services to engage with.

While the goals of encouraging healthy eating and improving general population health are admirable, the Tackling Obesity campaign highlights some of the problematic conceptions of health and agency that arise from neoliberal rationalities within health discourses, showing how these conceptions can lead to shame, blame and moral outrage. The campaign closely follows a neoliberal conception of health and citizenship, where individuals are positioned as self-actualizing with the unfettered capacity to make rational 'choices' about their behaviour and lifestyle, and are rendered personally responsible for their health status and body size as a result. Rather than recognizing 'the complex underlying causes of obesity [including] patho-physiological processes or a historical lack of effective public health policies … [or] genetic, environmental or socio-economic factors' that cause or contribute to obesity rates, the Tackling Obesity campaign individualizes the burden of blame, both in terms of who is responsible for a 'burden' on the health service and in terms of who should make more sensible 'choices' and 'swaps'.[49] Solving 'problems' related to obesity or excess weight is framed as simply 'a matter of future-oriented individual risk management'.[50]

One advertisement for the campaign shows an older man wearing hi-vis gear eating chopped fruit from a plastic tub, beside the tagline 'Healthy eating starts with simple swaps'. The idea, presumably, is that this individual has simply swapped an unhealthy snack for this healthier option. A new iteration of the Change4Life 'smart swap' campaign, these sorts of 'small changes' that individuals can make are at the heart of the new Tackling Obesity strategy. Boris Johnson is quoted as saying in the press release: 'Losing weight is hard but with some small changes we can all feel fitter and healthier.'[51] In reality, the 'simple swaps' that the campaign encourages are scaffolded by a range of socio-economic contingencies. Most people simply cannot afford to routinely buy the prohibitively expensive tubs of pre-chopped fruit that serve as the visual paradigm for a 'simple swap'.[52] By framing obesity as merely the result of an individual's 'choices', the Tackling Obesity campaign ignores the realities of those living with eating disorders or who have socio-economic or psycho-social constraints regarding the sorts of choices they can make about what foods to eat and when and where to exercise. Instead, the message is clear: not making the 'right' choices and swaps will in turn 'cost' others. Boris Johnson, again quoted in the press release, says, 'If we all do our bit, we can reduce our health risks and protect ourselves against coronavirus – as well as take pressure off the NHS.'[53]

In fact, the campaign explicitly and repeatedly emphasizes the *cost* associated with bodies with excess weight, reinforcing the idea that fat bodies are 'expensive', and, as a result, inherently unprofitable and unproductive.[54] The Tackling Obesity government strategy document states: 'tackling obesity would reduce pressure on doctors and nurses in the NHS, and free up their time to treat other sick and vulnerable patients'. It continues: 'we owe it to the NHS to move towards a healthier weight. Obesity puts pressure on our health service ... If all people who are overweight or living with obesity in the population lost just 2.5kg (one-third of a stone), it could save the NHS £105 million over the next 5 years'. It concludes: 'going into this winter, you can play your part to protect the NHS and save lives'.[55] In this way, individuals are exhorted to regulate their weight not only to benefit their own health but also, crucially, to minimize any 'burden' or 'cost' that they might pose to their healthcare systems as a result. This discourse positions individuals with excess weight as 'irresponsible' and 'inconsiderate'[56]; not only do their 'choices' negatively affect their individual health but they threaten the NHS, directly putting 'pressure' on doctors and taking resources away from 'sick and vulnerable patients'. Identifying those with a particular body size as putting a financial strain on the NHS, and potentially causing harm to others by taking up resources during the pandemic, immediately divides people into those who are deserving and those who are not, or those who should be 'praised' and those who can be stigmatized, shunned, shamed or 'mocked'.[57] Indeed, as a review of the campaign in *Nature Reviews* notes, the 'choice of language' in the Tackling Obesity Policy documents 'could be damaging as it encourages the blaming and shaming of people with overweight and obesity'.[58]

In fact, the campaign concretely demonstrates how implicit fat shaming – where 'heaping blame on shame' as a 'wilful political strategy' – is being operationalized within this public health effort. Not only are individuals with excess weight positioned in the discourse as blameworthy for being inconsiderate and irresponsible, literally *costing others*, they are also positioned as shame-worthy for seemingly lacking the willpower, rationality or social grace to make the right food and exercise choices, the 'simple swaps' or morning jogs, that will lead to weight loss. This shaming and blaming strategy is disappointing in light of the significant evidence in the public health literature showing that a focus on individual choices and using shame and blame strategies, whether implicit or explicit, in obesity campaigns is ineffective.[59] It is even more jarring considering the context within which the campaign was launched – immediately after a lengthy national lockdown, where most individuals were housebound, with both physical activity and food choices profoundly affected. Significant amounts of people reported weight gain during lockdown as a result of factors such as increased snacking, increased alcohol consumption, emotional eating to cope with stress and anxiety, difficulty getting to shops to get healthy food, less opportunity to exercise and being more sedentary in general.[60] In their report following a consultation with people living with obesity, Le Brocq et al. note:

> Lockdown presents substantial challenges to maintaining healthy behaviours for anyone; however, people living with obesity have often had years of battling with weight and experiencing feelings of guilt from perceived failure. Representatives in our consultation reported having a fear of weight gain during lockdown, related to the effect of anxiety on eating behaviours (often compounded by scrutiny from family members). For many, this fear related to stigma or shame and prevented them from exercising or shopping for food in ways that did not make them feel self-conscious. Lockdown has had a profound influence on self-efficacy, and increased episodes of secret eating or binge eating have been commonly reported within the Obesity UK support groups during this time.[61]

The idea in the Tackling Obesity campaign that individuals can simply 'choose' their food and exercise regimes is immediately undermined by the public health intervention (lockdown) which was rolled out to tackle the very impetus for the campaign (Covid-19). Participants in Grannell et al.'s study on the lived experience of people with obesity during Covid-19 reported how lockdown restrictions drastically curtailed opportunities for exercise, and that the fear of being more vulnerable to Covid-19 led to a significant psycho-social burden, while also limiting opportunities for exercise and having a negative impact on decision-making around food.[62]

The focus on individual choice and the 'cost' of excess weight, especially during a pandemic where many people are struggling with issues around health, stress and finances, sends a message which is largely counterproductive, leading to feelings of failure and shame related to weight stigma. In addition, these messages were not merely counterproductive but were possibly '*detrimental* for mental health, particularly for those with eating disorders', as Talbot and Branley-Bell note.[63] In their research, they show that social media users experienced the Tackling Obesity campaign as triggering 'disordered eating behaviours because of its fat-shaming approach, and focus on lower weight and calorie intake as equating to health'.[64] As Le Brocq et al. note, many people living with obesity experienced 'feelings of shame, a perception of being "less of a priority than any other condition", and a reluctance to seek help'.[65]

In addition, the roll-out of the Tackling Obesity initiative coincided exactly with the 'Eat Out to Help Out' initiative to stimulate economic growth, leading to inconsistent government messaging widely interpreted as 'hypocritical' and 'contradictory'.[66] Under this government scheme, members of the public were entitled to a 50 per cent discount, up to a value of £10, in restaurants during August 2020, and individuals were actively encouraged to eat out during the month, in order to boost the economy by supporting hospitality businesses. Many of the restaurants that signed up to take part were fast-food chains, such as KFC and McDonalds, which are directly implicated in weight gain and increases in obesity rates.[67] This mixed messaging further undermined public health efforts, leaving individuals feeling blameworthy and ashamed.

Despite public health evidence demonstrating that behaviour change approaches in health campaigns are not effective, the UK government's Tackling Obesity campaign emphasizes weight loss through individual responsibility, casting those who remain overweight as failures within a neoliberal framework that conceptualizes self-help as a choice that all can make to promote better overall health. Unsurprisingly, a recent study conducted by the Social Market Foundation has shown that the Tackling Obesity strategy has been 'largely ineffective'. The study stated that ministers placed too much emphasis on 'individual willpower and not enough on the environmental and economic aspects of obesity'.[68] Not only is the Tackling Obesity campaign both unproductive and ineffective, it is irresponsible in light of the available public health evidence on obesity and anti-obesity campaigns. Also irresponsible are official statements from the country's prime minister which suggest that 'small changes' are all that is needed for weight loss. Not only does this claim not match public health evidence, it creates a ripe atmosphere for government-sanctioned shame and blame for those who are not able to affect those 'changes' or for whom those 'changes' do not lead to perceptible weight loss. While Johnson boasted at the Conservative Party conference that he had lost the equivalent of twenty-six bags of sugar in weight,[69] many people living with obesity reported significant psycho-social harm as a result of the shaming and blaming rhetoric that was directed to those whose body size deemed them a potential 'cost' and 'burden' to others.

Despite claiming to be 'led by the science', a phrase used so often as to outgrow the meaning of its most frequent context (in debates over restrictions to everyday life), the UK government's interventions on obesity and Covid-19 went against the grain of the vast majority of credible research on shame, stigma and public health design, as well as how members of targeted populations frequently report that campaigns which simplify and individualize the challenge make them feel. The government-led Foresight report, for example, highlighted in 2007 that obesity is complex, multi-faceted and not reducible to simple solutions or representations as a matter of individual willpower.[70] Criticisms of past campaigns have asserted that they actively cause harm (and do little or no good) by stigmatizing the intended recipients of their messaging, and WHO guidelines on weight bias and obesity stigma clearly state that 'narratives around obesity may contribute to weight bias by oversimplifying the causes of obesity and implying that easy solutions will lead to quick and sustainable results ("eat less, be more active"), thereby setting unrealistic expectations and masking the difficult challenges people with obesity can face in changing behaviour'.[71]

More important to the UK government than getting this response 'right', that is, by absorbing insights from research and activism on shame and stigma in public health and building them into their pandemic messaging, their shaming focus on individual choice reaffirmed a series of logics which are crucial to the stories they want to tell about inequality, responsibility, health and citizenship. Thus, fat shaming becomes a knowing political act which continually asserts a neoliberal understanding of health and success as the result of competitive choices and acts of consumption, to which everyone, in theory, has access.[72] Roberta Bivins notes how, in the 'common sense' of post-war Britain, 'only individuals could control their weight'; this is the common sense that present-day policy promotes, with overweight people as its intentional victims.[73] In the following chapter, we explore how a frequent emphasis on common sense in government rhetoric made further space for shame, reducing complex experiences and contexts to simplified equations of individual 'sense' and choice.

Notes

1. Luke Harding, Rowena Mason, Dan Sabbagh, Mattha Busby, Denis Campbell and Owen Bowcott, '"Boris Johnson and Coronavirus: The Inside Story of His Illness"', *The Guardian*, 17 April 2020, 13.31 BST. https://www.theguardian.com/world/2020/apr/17/boris-johnson-and-coronavirus-inside-story-illness.

2. Rowena Mason, 'Boris Johnson Still Has Covid-19 Symptoms and May Stay in Isolation', *The Guardian*, 2 April 2020, 14.48 BST. https://www.theguardian.com/politics/2020/apr/02/boris-johnson-shows-covid-19-symptoms-still-and-may-stay-in-isolation.

3. Luke Harding et al., 'Boris Johnson and Coronavirus'.

4. Luke Harding et al., 'Boris Johnson and Coronavirus'.

5. Luke Harding et al., 'Boris Johnson and Coronavirus'.

6. Simon Murphy, 'Boris Johnson Waved Thanks to NHS Staff as He Left Intensive Care', *The Guardian*, 10 April 2020, 16.11 BST. https://www.theguardian.com/politics/2020/apr/10/boris-johnson-father-stanley-tells-relief-pm-leaves-intensive-care.

7. '"I was too fat": Boris Johnson Launches UK Obesity Reduction Drive', *The Guardian*, 27 July 2020, 11.22 BST, video. https://www.theguardian.com/world/video/2020/jul/27/i-was-too-fat-boris-johnson-launches-uk-obesity-reduction-drive-video.

8. '"I was too fat": Boris Johnson Explains His "nasty" Brush with Covid', 6 October 2020, video. https://www.youtube.com/watch?v=EyPMIOGGXMs.

9. Public Health England, 'Excess Weight Can Increase Risk of Serious Illness and Death from COVID-19', Public Health England Press Release, 25 July 2020. https://www.gov.uk/government/news/excess-weight-can-increase-risk-of-serious-illness-and-death-from-covid-19.

10. Public Health England, 'Excess Weight Can Increase Risk of Serious Illness and Death from COVID-19'.

11. Public Health England, 'Excess Weight Can Increase Risk of Serious Illness and Death from COVID-19'.

12. '"I was too fat": Boris Johnson Launches UK Obesity Reduction Drive', video.

13. Kathleen LeBesco, 'Fat Panic and the New Morality', in *Against Health*, eds. Jonathan M. Metzl and Anna Kirkland (New York: New York University Press, 2015), 72–82.

14. Roberta Bivins, 'Weighing on Us All? Quantification and Cultural Responses to Obesity in NHS Britain', *History of Science* vol. 58:2 (2020), 216–42. https://doi.org/10.1177/0073275319842965.

15. Martha Kirby, 'Too Much of a Good Thing? Society, Affluence and Obesity in Britain, 1940–1970', *eSharp* vol. 18 (2012), 44–63, 50. https://www.gla.ac.uk/media/Media_228377_smxx.pdf.

16. Kirby, 'Too Much of a Good Thing?', 56.

17. Kirby, 'Too Much of a Good Thing?', 55–6.

18. Bivins, 'Weighing on Us All?', 227.

19. Jane Hand, '"Look After Yourself": Visualising Obesity as a Public Health Concern in 1970s and 1980s Britain', in *Balancing the Self: Medicine, Politics and the Regulation of Health in the Twentieth Century*, eds. Mark Jackson and Martin D. Moore (Manchester: Manchester University Press, 2020), 112.

20. Paul Baker et al., 'Changing Frames of Obesity in the UK Press 2008–2017', *Social Science & Medicine* vol. 264 (2020), 2–9. https://doi.org/10.1016/j.socscimed.2020.113403.#.

21. Bivins, 'Weighing on Us all?', 235, 238–9.

22. Baker et al., 'Changing Frames of Obesity in the UK Press 2008–2017', 6.

23. Martin D. Moore, 'Historicising "containment and delay": COVID-19, the NHS and High-Risk Patients' [version 1; peer review: 2 approved], *Wellcome Open Research* vol. 5:130 (2020). https://doi.org/10.12688/wellcomeopenres.15962.1.

24. Sue McGregor, 'Neoliberalism and Health Care', *International Journal of Consumer Studies* vol. 25:2 (2001), 82–9.

25. David Sturgeon, 'The Business of the NHS: The Rise and Rise of Consumer Culture and Commodification in the Provision of Healthcare Services', *Critical Social Policy* vol. 34:3 (2014), 408–9.

26. Sturgeon, 'The Business of the NHS', 414.

27. Tanisha Jemma Rose Spratt, 'Understanding "Fat Shaming" in a Neoliberal Era: Performativity, Healthism and the Uk's "Obesity Epidemic"', *Feminist Theory* (2021), 1–16. Published online first: DOI: 10.1177/14647001211048300.

28. Ted Schrecker and Clare Bambra, *How Politics Makes Us Sick: Neoliberal Epidemics* (Basingstoke: Palgrave Macmillan, 2015), 22.

29. Hannele Harjunen, *Neoliberal Bodies and the Gendered Fat Body* (London: Routledge, 2017), 5.

30. Spratt, 'Understanding "Fat Shaming" in a Neoliberal Era', 6.

31. Amy Erdman Farrell, *Fat Shame: Stigma and the Fat Body in American Culture* (New York: New York University Press, 2011), 4, 5.

32. Harjunen, *Neoliberal Bodies and the Gendered Fat Body*, 6.

33. Farrell, *Fat Shame, 2*, 5.

34. Alexandra Brewis and Amber Wutich, *Lazy, Crazy and Disgusting: Stigma and the Undoing of Global Health* (Baltimore: Johns Hopkins University Press, 2019), 78.

35. Harjunen, *Neoliberal Bodies and the Gendered Fat Body*, 5.

36. Spratt, 'Understanding "Fat Shaming" in a Neoliberal Era', 4.

37. Spratt, 'Understanding "Fat Shaming" in a Neoliberal Era', 1.

38. Spratt, 'Understanding "Fat Shaming" in a Neoliberal Era', 4.

39. The discussion of the Tackling Obesity campaign that follows is partly drawn from Dolezal's discussion in the co-authored article: Tanisha Spratt and Luna Dolezal, 'Fat Shaming under Neoliberalism and Covid-19: Examining the UK's "Tackling Obesity" Campaign', OSF Preprints, 13 July 2021, https://doi.org/10.31219/osf.io/2ymun.

40. Cyrielle Caussy, Florent Wallet, Martine Laville and Emmanuel Disse,'Obesity is Associated with Severe Forms of Covid-19', Obesity vol. 28 (2020), 1175, https://doi.org/10.1002/oby.22842.

41. Department of Health & Social Care, 'Tackling Obesity: Empowering Adults and Children to Live Healthier Lives', Department of Health & Social Care Policy Paper, 27 July 2020. https://www.gov.uk/government/publications/tackling-obesity-government-strategy/tackling-obesity-empowering-adults-and-children-to-live-healthier-lives.

42. Alan Glasper, 'Obesity Levels and COVID-19: The Government's Mission', Journal of Nursing vol. 29:18 (2020), 1082.

43. Glasper, 'Obesity Levels and COVID-19'; '"I was too fat": Boris Johnson Launches UK Obesity Reduction Drive', video.

44. '"I was too fat": Boris Johnson Launches UK Obesity Reduction Drive', video.

45. '"I was too fat": Boris Johnson Launches UK Obesity Reduction Drive', video.

46. BBC News, 'Boris in Row over Jamie Remarks' (2006), 3 October. http://news.bbc.co.uk/1/hi/uk_politics/5404438.stm.

47. Public Health England, 'Swap while You Shop: New Campaign Launched to Get Families Making Healthy Swaps in January', Public Health England Press Release (2014), https://www.gov.uk/government/news/swap-while-you-shop-new-campaign-launched-to-get-families-making-healthy-swaps-in-january.

48. Department of Health & Social Care, 'Tackling Obesity: Empowering Adults and Children to Live Healthier Lives'.

49. 'UK policy targeting obesity during a pandemic — the right approach?', Nature Reviews Endocrinology 16, 609 (2020). https://doi.org/10.1038/s41574-020-00420-x.

50. Jane Mulderrig, 'Reframing Obesity: A Critical Discourse Analysis of the UK's First Social Marketing Campaign', Critical Policy Studies vol. 11:4 (2017), 457.

51. Department of Health and Social Care, 'New Obesity Strategy Unveiled as Country Urged to Lose Weight to Beat Coronavirus (COVID-19) and Protect the NHS'.

52. Rachel Cooke, 'Why Boris Johnson's New Anti-Obesity Strategy makes me reach for the Chocolate', The Guardian, 17:00 BST, 15 August 2020. https://www.theguardian.com/food/2020/aug/15/why-boris-johnsons-new-anti-obesity-strategy-makes-me-reach-for-the-chocolate?CMP=Share_iOSApp_Other.

53. Department of Health and Social Care, 'New Obesity Strategy Unveiled as Country Urged to Lose Weight to Beat Coronavirus (COVID-19) and Protect the NHS'.

54. Harjunen, *Neoliberal Bodies and the Gendered Fat Body*, 6.

55. Department of Health & Social Care, 'Tackling Obesity: Empowering Adults and Children to Live Healthier Lives.'

56. Spratt, 'Understanding "Fat Shaming" in a Neoliberal Era', 6.

57. Farrell, *Fat Shame*, 5.

58. 'UK Policy Targeting Obesity during a Pandemic – the Right Approach?', *Nature Reviews Endocrinology* vol. 16:609 (2020). https://doi.org/10.1038/s41574-020-00420-x.

59. Brewis and Wutich, *Lazy, Crazy and Disgusting*.

60. Zeigler, Z. et al., 'Self-Quarantine and Weight Gain Related Risk Factors during the COVID-19 Pandemic', *Obesity Research & Clinical Practice* vol. 14 (2020), 210–6; COVID Symptom Study, 'The Silent Pandemic: How Lockdown Is Affecting Future Health', 2020. https://covid.joinzoe.com/post/lockdown-weight-gain; BBC Food, 'Lockdown and Weight Gain – Should You Worry?', (2020). https://www.bbc.co.uk/food/articles/lockdown_health_tips.

61. S. Le Brocq, K. Clare, M. Bryant, K. Roberts and A. A. Tahrani, 'Obesity and COVID-19: A Call for Action from People Living with Obesity', *The Lancet Diabetes & Endocinology* vol. 8:8 (2020), 653.

62. Andrew Grannell, Carel W. le Roux and Deirdre McGillicuddy, '"I am terrified of something happening to me": The Lived Experience of People with Obesity during the COVID-19 Pandemic', *Clinical Obesity* vol. 10:6 (2020), e12406.

63. Talbot and Branley-Bell. '#BetterHealth', 3.

64. Talbot and Branley-Bell. '#BetterHealth', 3.

65. Le Brocq et al., 'Obesity and COVID-19', 653.

66. Talbot and Branley-Bell, '#BetterHealth', 4.

67. Janet Currie, Stefano Della Vigna, Enrico Moretti and Vikram Pathania, 'The Effect of Fast Food Restaurants on Obesity and Weight Gain', *American Economic Journal* vol. 2:3 (2010), 32–63.

68. Social Market Foundation, 'Covid Warnings Aren't an Effective Obesity Strategy', 2020. https://www.smf.co.uk/covid-warnings-arent-an-effective-obesity-strategy/.

69. '"I was too fat": Boris Johnson Explains His "nasty" Brush with Covid', 6 October 2020, video. https://www.youtube.com/watch?v=EyPMIOGGXMs.

70. Baker et al., 'Changing Frames of Obesity in the UK Press 2008–2017', 8; Foresight, 'Tackling Obesities: Future Choices – Project report', Government Office for Science, 17 October 2007. https://www.gov.uk/government/publications/reducing-obesity-future-choices.

71. Joanne A Rathbone, Tegan Cruwys, and Jolanda Jetten, 'Non-Stigmatising Alternatives to Anti-Obesity Public Health Messages: Consequences for Health Behaviour and Well-Being', *Journal of Health Psychology* (March 2021).

https://doi.org/10.1177/1359105321999705; World Health Organisation Regional Office for Europe, *Weight Bias and Obesity Stigma: Considerations for the WHO European Region* (Copenhagen: WHO, 2017). https://www.euro.who.int/__data/assets/pdf_file/0017/351026/WeightBias.pdf.

72. Stuart Hall and Alan O'Shea, 'Common-sense Neoliberalism', *Soundings: A journal of politics and culture* vol. 55 (2013), 8–24, 12.

73. Bivins, 'Weighing on Us All?', 228.

CHAPTER 5
GOOD SOLID BRITISH COMMON SENSE: SHAME AND SURVEILLANCE IN EVERYDAY LIFE

11 May 2020. Boris Johnson stands up in House of Commons to give a statement on the government's ongoing Covid-19 strategy. He advocates strongly for a change in guidance, from the 'stay at home' message pursued through lockdown to a more abstract injunction, 'stay alert'. Members of Parliament quiz him on the reasons for the change, whether it is informed by scientific evidence, indeed what the new command even means. Blustering that the new guidance is 'perfectly obvious', that the public 'understand exactly what we are trying to do', Johnson's responses return, time and again, to the idea of 'common sense'. Indeed, in the course of his statement he offers perhaps the best-known (and most widely critiqued) example of what the Government meant by common sense:

> But let us be clear: everybody understands what we are trying to do together. We are working together as a country to obey the social distancing rules, which everybody understands. The British people understand that this is the moment for the whole country to come together, obey those rules, and apply common sense in their application of them … I know that the British public will continue to help the police, and everybody, to enforce the rules, get the reproduction rate down, and get this disease even further under control, by continuing to apply good, solid, British common sense.[1]

In the government's messaging on public behaviour during the pandemic, the grey areas between law and advice were frequently regulated by appeals to common sense.[2] Johnson's emphasis on common sense – and the partial de-escalation of quarantine measures it sought to clarify – was met with a range of criticisms, some of which set out to unpick common sense as a rhetorical device and political idea.[3] These critiques drew largely on pre-existing philosophical and sociological reckonings with common sense, at times highlighting the role that common sense discourses play in the continuation of neoliberal logics and anti-expert populism.[4] Johnson prefixed 'common sense' with anchoring or 'guiding' words such as 'good', 'solid', and 'British'; these have long been observed as key to the ways that common sense is framed and naturalized in a misleading language of instinct, popular knowledge, and authenticity.[5]

In the context of new admonitions to 'stay alert', Johnson's words were also interpreted as an exercise in deflecting shame and saving face. Both in contemporary political and academic criticism, and in what could be described as the 'good sense' observations of some 'ordinary' members of the public, they seemed to represent a deliberate slippage of responsibility for the course of the pandemic away from the decisions and shortcomings of the state, and towards individual behaviour, perception and reasoning. While common sense itself is usually defined as a collective social and cultural achievement, its absence or lack is figured as a personal failing, and a potential source of blame and shame.[6] Johnson's invocation of common sense helped to reproduce an imagined community with longer historical roots, deferring expertise to an implicitly nationalistic popular wisdom; simultaneously, it framed the public it sought to flatter for the foreseeably negative outcomes of a market-driven return to business as usual.[7] It perpetuated, therefore, what Stuart Hall and Alan O'Shea describe as the 'structural consequences' of common-sense neoliberalism: 'the individualisation of everyone, the privatisation of public troubles and the requirement to make competitive choices at every turn'.[8] When he stated 'that the British public will continue to help the police, and everybody, to enforce the rules', Johnson gestured to the raised public stakes of pandemic common sense, as a matter of both individual and collective vigilance. At a moment where expected behaviour was particularly unclear, members of the public were invited to apply the nebulous and subjective principles of common sense not just in their own decision-making but to the actions of relatives, friends, neighbours, acquaintances, colleagues and strangers.[9]

This chapter interrogates common sense as public health policy, situating the individualization of responsibility for Covid-19 within longer and deeper critiques of common sense as a political and cultural idea. In the process, it draws focus to an under-acknowledged consequence of poor public health policy: the increased burden of shame. Making use of Mass Observation testimonies from the spring and summer of 2020, the chapter explores how respondents deployed and contested government narratives on common sense, and how public health messaging which sought to save face for the government made unnecessary space for guilt, blame and shame. Applying common sense to each other's actions erases the complex histories and contexts which frame and condition behaviour, knowledge and 'choice', privileging a shaming accountability to a conceptual phantom which, as one Mass Observer noted, 'varies from one person to another and means completely different things and behaviour'.[10] As an emotion with extensive consequences for behaviour, shame can also prompt people to act in ways which seem counter to common sense, but which are consistent with logics of avoidance or concealment.[11] What seems like common sense is frequently incompatible with the lived realities of inequality, poverty or suffering, failing to reckon with other kinds of survival made necessary by a structural inattention to the economic, psychological and relational fallout of the virus.[12]

Common sense

Mass Observation participants interpreted 'stay alert' and 'good solid British common sense' in different ways. For respondents who were already broadly critical of the government, these pronouncements felt like a 'dangerous blame game', a means to 'blame the public for any problems' or, in a different formulation, of 'blaming others for failures'.[13] Others were less critical of intention but sceptical of common sense as a public health response, and anxious about the consequences. Presciently, one seventy-year-old former secretary observed that the country had entered a 'dangerous situation where eventually the public was just told to "use your common sense." This, I am sure, will lead to a further spike in the numbers of positive tests and deaths when presumably everything will be locked down again'.[14] The respondent who complained that common sense 'varies from one person to another and means completely different things and behaviour' concluded that 'we really can't be trusted at the moment to get it right'.[15] These two responses probed the limitations of common sense as a strategy for viral containment, but they leaned on relatively predictable and well-trodden observations – what we might term common sense about common sense – at the same time; the flaw in the government's approach, implicitly, is that common sense is 'in reality' neither commonly held (widely and evenly dispersed among the population) nor held in common (the consistent product of genuine consensus). This mode of critique leaves the category of common sense conceptually intact; in this respect, it echoes the philosopher Stanley Rosen's aphorism that 'common sense is not honoured but betrayed when we assign it a task which it cannot fulfil'.[16]

In other Mass Observation testimonies, common sense was a straightforward and meaningful resource, a practical set of principles which was made use of (usually by the writer), or ignored (usually by the subject of the writer's judgement, ire, or scorn). Some respondents broadly accepted the government's individualization of blame, complaining that 'it has taken a while for everyone to apply common sense', or asserting that 'people should take responsibility for themselves and have some common sense'.[17] Common sense could also be repurposed as a mode of political critique. Across her responses to two directives, one Mass Observer painted a vivid and familiar picture of pandemic television viewing:

'It seems that we have all been shouting at our TV's going "NO, we need to do X Y Z." Things that seem obvious common sense were just not applied.'[18]
'We watch the news a lot and shout at the telly because what seems common sense to us (face masks and quarantine for people arriving in the country) are simply not happening.'[19]

While the second comment clearly described the behaviour of the respondent and her household, the 'we' in 'it seems that we have all been shouting' is far more encompassing, setting a broad popular common sense in tension with the actions of the government. For all of the evidence and expertise available to them, they were failing to take measures which were 'obvious' to the public at large.[20]

The UK government's framing of pandemic behaviour in terms of common sense – and the clear diversity of public responses even among a handful of testimonies – raises vital questions over what common sense is, where it comes from and how it works. For the sake of brevity, we divide literatures on common sense into two loose camps. On the one hand, we have scholarship which takes the fundamental idea of common sense at face value, and attempts to define and understand it as a knowable cultural and social resource. On the other – and particularly in literature which responds politically to ideological changes in the UK, America and Western Europe in the final decades of the twentieth century – we have a reckoning with common sense as a means of shaping and policing the boundaries of what is or isn't 'possible', 'reasonable' or 'sane', of imposing a particular set of (more recently, neoliberal) logics on political (and personal) behaviour and attributing them to the wisdom and sense of 'common' people. Each of these lenses on common sense can help us to understand why it failed as a public health response, resulting in increased transmission, higher mortality and morbidity rates, prolonged periods of quarantine, and unnecessary and preventable experiences of shame.

If we approach common sense – as the government has repeatedly invited the public to – as both a tangible individual characteristic and a universally accessible fund, then what is the shared (or common) meaning of the term? According to the historian Sophia Rosenfeld, a (relatively) recognizable iteration of common sense emerged from philosophical debates on perception and realism in the eighteenth century, as part of the scientific and intellectual flourishing collectively known as the Scottish Enlightenment. In the specific political context of the eighteenth and nineteenth centuries, common sense was increasingly valorized as 'a new "epistemic authority"' with the potential to go head to head with considerably more established forms of authority, including history, law, custom, faith, logic, and reason, especially when it came to matters of social or moral life'.[21] In theory, common sense is common because it is available to everyone, whether they use it or not.[22] For Pierre Bourdieu, common sense is 'a stock of self-evidences shared by all, which, within the limits of a social universe, ensures a primordial consensus on the meaning of the world, a set of tacitly accepted commonplaces which make confrontation, dialogue, competition and even conflict possible'.[23] Bourdieu explains how common sense structures a collective frame of reference to 'think the world', even as subjective valuations of agreed-on terms diverge: 'thus the same freedom of manners may be seen by some as "shameless", impolite, rude, and by others as "unaffected", simple, unpretentious, natural'.[24]

Explicitly lacking in intellectual sophistication or complexity, the 'stock of self-evidences' which comprise common sense concern themselves specifically with what Anna Wierzbicka terms 'the question of what to think in a particular situation so as to know – and know quickly – what to do and what not to do there and then'.[25] In her work on the historical origins of common sense, Rosenfeld sets up a long historical tension between this supposedly 'infallible, instinctive sense of what is right and true, born of or nurtured by day-to-day experience in the world', and the 'judgements and knowledge of a minority of establishment insiders', expanded in the recent past 'to include, varyingly, intellectuals, scientists, financiers, lawyers, journalists, power brokers, politicians, and other overeducated, elite pretenders, as well as foreigners and outliers of different kinds'.[26] She reads it, therefore, as organizing and subsuming many of the same kinds of anti-establishment anger which would later be harnessed and directed by populist political projects.

By invoking a broad, anti-expert populism, the rhetoric of common sense seems to distance it from technical evidence and expertise, while using these as important sources of practical knowledge, which sediment down into culturally, historically, and politically inflected insights and impressions about 'how the world works'.[27] Every institution involved in the reproduction and transmission of knowledge plays a part in these processes, with the media as particularly significant intermediaries and gatekeepers.[28] Common sense and diffused or disseminated expertise, however, are not the same. Even if we take common sense as a meaningful and internally consistent idea, there are deep fissures between how it is purported to operate and how it has been deployed as a public health measure during Covid-19. Probing the boundaries of common sense in the mid-1960s, Rosen described it as 'the capacity to deal successfully with the commonly accessible world'. Common sense is limited in its capacity to offer universal answers, he argued, because 'the world of common experience is not an objective, fully defined entity', but 'murky and ambiguous' instead.[29]

During Covid-19, a 'commonly accessible world' of pandemic common sense was unavailable for three reasons. In the first instance, as Rosen implied, such a resource is probably always elusive, whatever the context or subject of application. In the second instance, the rapid and shifting flow of events, information, advice and legal requirements has been far too frenetic and uneven to allow anything resembling common sense to emerge. Discussing Bourdieu's understanding of common sense, Robert Holton explains how an 'objective social crisis' can 'put the practices of common sense into question, thereby undermining its self-evidence ... the common sense of yesterday becomes inapplicable today'. The historical and social production of common sense responds to alterations in conditions and contexts, but this is not an immediate or uniform process.[30] If something like pandemic common sense is possible, therefore, it might be produced by long social and cultural experiences of quarantine, distancing, mask-wearing and handwashing, for example, but not by expectations about when or why these measures should be introduced or discontinued, or how policy and scientific data should be interpreted. What stands in for common sense instead is a loose and disparate series of personal judgements, impressions and apprehensions, framed by a subjective emotional and intellectual digestion of evidence on risk, and filtered in turn through pre-existing prejudices, tendencies and feelings over personal and collective safety and responsibility. Applying common sense, here, is reduced to individualized decisions over whether or not to abide by earlier public health instructions and injunctions, newly tempered into guidelines and advice. With parallels to the discussion of pandemic shaming in Chapter 1, injunctions to use 'common sense' replaced a formal disciplinary system (police action, legal sanction) with an informal one (shared responsibility for the course of the pandemic and the potential for public or interpersonal shame).

In the third instance, the inaccessibility and unevenness of public health communication across the pandemic has further militated against the emergence of anything like common sense as a viable collective resource. Other chapters in this book have discussed how specific groups and communities were targeted with campaigns that increased their burden of shame, making them less likely to engage with public health messaging (see Chapter 4), or how longer cycles of shame and abandonment were reproduced by conscious decisions over where, how and what to communicate, with the myth of 'hard to reach' populations deflecting shame from institutions to the people they fail to successfully engage (see Chapter 3). Research into the pandemic experiences of people with dementia, for example, further punctures the suggestion of a 'commonly accessible' sense, with unclear and confusing guidance limiting respondents' participation in society and 'contributing to their shrinking worlds'.[31] As one testimony put it, 'if I was living on my own, I would have no idea what was going on because it was so airy-fairy and common sense here'.[32]

These experiences support Rosenfeld's observation that common sense 'works in practice to create new forms of exclusion', constructing imagined communities defined by common sense at the expense of specific out-groups. These include people with views considered 'superstitious, marginal, or deluded', or 'overly abstract, specialized, or dogmatic', as well as people whose ability to navigate the world in ways consistent with the logic of common sense is hindered by structural ableism or inequality.[33] There are compelling reasons to approach the counterintuitive divisiveness of common sense as a deliberate political aim, and mistrust its rhetorical deployment in the context of Covid-19 as a sincere policy which – for the reasons detailed above – happened to fail. As a cynical exercise in delegitimizing public health expertise, it shifted culpability away from the state and nourished an idea which serves specific political purposes in the way that it shapes and conditions ideological discourses.[34] As Holton puts it:

The world's meaning must continually be reaffirmed and/or reconstructed as common sense precisely because it is a historical world constantly open to challenge and to struggle, because the possibility continues to exist that its meaning may slip away, because it is in the interest of some that certain aspects of its meaning should slip away and be replaced with other meanings.[35]

The meanings that slip away, in this context, relate to how government decisions and omissions have resulted in catastrophic outcomes for the UK population, and the well-evidenced fact that these have not been equally borne or distributed. Reconfiguring public health as common sense replaces these inconvenient and shameful meanings with a neoliberal emphasis on individual agency and culpability, removing shame from state harms and relocating it to the victims.[36]

Even before neoliberalism fell into widespread use as a term of critique, common sense had been identified as an idea consistent with the logics of me-first individualism. For Rosen, common sense imposes a hierarchy of outcomes, 'in which self-preservation, and then a secure and even comfortable self-preservation, predominate'. Injunctions to use common sense, therefore, become 'do what is best for you', which in turn becomes 'protect yourself' or 'get what you can'.[37] Through this logical creep, common sense actively works against notions of communal solidarity and safety, both in response to the pandemic and in wider ideological terms. Critics of the government's recent uses of common sense trace a line in conservative rhetoric from William Hague's 'Common Sense Revolution' in 2001, through David Cameron's justification of austerity policies as 'common sense for the common good' in the early 2010s, and Jacob Rees-Mogg's speculation over whether common sense might have saved the victims of the Grenfell Tower fire, to 'common sense' criticisms of (often invented) EU restrictions, and the earthy pragmatism of pronouncements on 'getting Brexit done'.[38] A political and social world organized by common sense, in short, is one which suits a specific Conservative ideological and electoral agenda.[39]

In the Covid-19 pandemic, the politicized invocation of common sense is one of many indications that this agenda is prioritized above positive epidemiological outcomes. Even when common sense was used to critique the state – as was the case in some of the Mass Observation testimonies discussed above – this does not necessarily imply a break with government intentions. A long ambivalence in the Conservative Party's relationship with expertise has frequently allowed for the representation of particular politicians as soothsayers of a broadly defined popular will; appeals to common sense help destabilize rival sources of narrative authority, in a way that permits dissent within distinct and manageable parameters.[40] Public uses of common sense as a basis to dispute government decisions, lapses or missteps, therefore, are an acceptable side product of a calculating political project. The stickiness or slipperiness of shame in relation to power differentials ensures that shame over shortfalls in common sense primarily lands in ways that burden 'common' people rather than politicians (see Chapter 1).

Common shame

In one Mass Observation day diary for 12 May 2020, the day after Johnson's reference to 'good British common sense', the author brought common sense and potential shame into close proximity: 'me and my husband have been out and about as normal – though you have to lie to friends as they wouldn't approve at all. We've just used common sense rather than blindly follow what the government says'.[41] The government's use of common sense as a device to shift responsibility for the pandemic onto individual behaviour contained a clear invitation for members of the public to police the actions of others. This was formalized in new infrastructures of reporting, for example through the creation of an online portal on www.police.uk to 'tell us about a possible breach of coronavirus (Covid-19) measures'.[42] In September 2020, the Home Office minister Kit Malthouse made it clear that people should call a non-emergency police number if they witnessed others gathering in groups of more than six, with the home secretary, Priti Patel, emphasizing that she would personally report her own neighbours if they broke with government guidance.[43] While many doubtless felt less comfortable resorting to the apparatus of criminal justice than Patel, this encouragement of mutual surveillance, regulated by common sense, resulted in an informal – but no less affecting – atmosphere of judgement and shame.

Mass Observers frequently reproduced shaming narratives over 'idiotic' behaviour. Only one of hundreds of testimonies openly admitted to having potentially caused shame, and discussed stigma (around failing to wear masks) as a favourable outcome; even though the immediate impetus to cause shame is usually self-righteous, practices of shaming can be shameful (and themselves targets of shame backlashes) on later reflection.[44] Discussing the behaviour of other shoppers, the author wrote that:

the front of the queue were so close to each other they could have cuddled. In my bit of the queue I had to ask the person behind me to move to 2 metres away. She did comply but looked angry (or maybe shamed?) Why are people behaving so badly? They clearly think the guidance does not apply to them or that they can't get sick or make others sick.

Relieved that indoor face masks were about to become compulsory, they noted, 'I guess we have to wait for it [not wearing a mask] to be as socially stigmatising as smoking in public places? What a shame.'[45]

Other testimonies merely confirmed the mind-set which underpinned rarer instances of direct confrontation. People who failed to follow guidelines or apply common sense were 'covidiots', a 'Covid idiot' (see Chapter 1), or 'gross idiots'.[46] Only one testimony implied any real disquiet at public shaming as a widespread social practice during the pandemic:

One of the weirdest things about Lockdown is how much certain people seemed to be enjoying it. I had people on Facebook taking videos of people walking down the street and in the park and ranting about how dreadful these people were for going outside. There were people who kept typing 'STAY THE FUCK HOME!!!' There was a thread on Mumsnet which basically consisted of a bunch of women moaning about how much we hated Lockdown and every so often someone would come onto it to tell everybody how Wrong and Selfish we were to complain.[47]

The effects of these processes are legible in other Mass Observation testimonies. In detailing their everyday lives during the pandemic, some respondents discussed acute experiences of shame, instances where they felt hyper-visible and vulnerable to judgement. In the words of Mass Observers, we can read how guilt and shame actively narrowed social and relational worlds, and created logics of shame-avoidance which frequently went against the grain of both 'common sense' and different kinds of pandemic survival. Some responses described how guilt altered and compromised experiences of being out in public, which can be lifelines for many even under non-pandemic circumstances:

'These days, I try to not to go out at all if I can help it. I can't stand all the social judgement about where we should stand.'

'Queues felt as though there was an atmosphere of collective guilt at being out of the house - nobody spoke to one another.'[48]

Particularly for people with long experiences of loneliness, brief exchanges with familiar faces or friendly strangers can be a vital source of relational sustenance, often overlooked by an emphasis on deep and confiding relationships in academic literatures.[49] Freighted with guilt and the potential for shaming transgression, these small but significant connections are more or less impossible to replace, in the way that established relationships can be sustained online or over the telephone. Apprehension over shame in public spaces, therefore, can be understood as an important determinant of pandemic isolation, with overlapping physical and mental consequences. Acting here in opposition to relational health, shame could also interfere with measures aimed at disrupting viral transmission; one Mass Observer wrote about a loaded cultural valuation of face masks as signifiers of illness rather than prevention, at least in the early days of the pandemic; in this context, her mother had written 'that she does not want me to wear a mask for fear that the neighbours will think she has the virus.'[50]

Two more responses bear repeating at length, for their close and nuanced representation of difficult experiences of shame and surveillance. In the first, a day diary from 12 May 2020, a runner recalls a jarring encounter with two older walkers:

I go to pass by them, and momentarily catch onto their eyes. They both throw me quick glances as they hastily shuffle onto the side of the pavement away from me, despite already having enough room to pass by. Then they are behind me, gone. I try to place my focus back onto my breathing as I continue forward but that image of those two pairs of judging eyes imprints itself onto my vision. "Is what I'm doing wrong?" I think to myself... I have been so used to passers-by ignoring me, so used to them pretending that I'm just not there, that it is astonishingly weird to see them react to my presence as I run past them, for them to simply acknowledge my existence. In this strange era of suspicion and sensitivity, it seems that no one is invisible, not even the runners.[51]

Shame, in this instance, was located in the 'astonishingly weird' transformation from an implicitly welcome invisibility to unwished-for and uncomfortable scrutiny and judgement, a transformation which left an emotional 'imprint' far outlasting the fleeting temporality of the physical encounter. Their common sense interpretation of what they should and shouldn't do had come into dissonant conflict with that of the two walkers; the runner felt judged, and this led them to a shamed reconsideration of behaviour which was legal and responsible, and which had positive consequences for their physical and mental wellbeing.

In the second response, a justified feeling of being surveilled by neighbours caused one respondent to retreat from his garden, fall into 'odd' habits, and reproduce the same kinds of judgemental behaviour which had led to his own distress:

> During the early days of lockdown a friend wanted to come round, I thought it would be ok, as I have a big garden, she could keep her distance, I provided anti bacteria gel, when my neighbour climbed up on his small roof where his twin six year olds normally sit, and he challenged me about the rules and did they not apply to me? My friend left quietly, I was stunned by this, these are people I have known for nine years … I really felt like I was being policed, my reaction was to shut down, I kept the front room curtain closed, I stayed away from the front of the house when I knew the family next door were in their garden, I removed myself from the back garden when I knew the mother was out the back with her kids … I found my own behaviour became odd, watching them from the top front window, breaking rules, not keeping the social distance, I realized this craziness, it was sending me bonkers, as now I wasn't able to really be who I am.[52]

While the respondent makes no explicit mention of common sense, its logic is threaded through the first part of his testimony; in his admission that he 'thought it would be ok', and in his subsequent list of mitigating circumstances to an imagined reader. This way of framing the episode is a clear appeal to common sense, uniting us in the judgement that his behaviour was safe – if not legal – and that his neighbours' reaction was irrational, absurd, and over the top. What emerges from this account is an unsettling description of alienation and estrangement, both from his neighbours and from an abstract notion of an authentic self. Even more strikingly, he situated a new and uncharacteristic tendency to watch and judge as a crucial component of these broken relational bonds. His neighbours' attempts to shame him simultaneously dissipated his trust, and held them (as potential hypocrites) to pristine and impossible standards of behaviour, which of course they could never live up to.

In this testimony, the respondent begins to judge others for their transgression of public health advice, not from a position of self-righteousness or relative power but from an abject position of vulnerability, unwanted visibility and shame. The sudden and painful discovery that his common sense was not common at all but subject instead to shaming scrutiny and confrontation caused him to temporarily become someone who might in turn cast shame: a subjectivity he found difficult and unrecognizable. Bringing important questions of structural harm into sharp relief, his testimony – and many of the others discussed here – marks some of the serious relational consequences of policies which made needless room for shame rather than addressing it as a serious barrier to collective health.

This chapter has focused in part on 'common shame', instances of shame around Covid-19 made possible by lack of clarity on government guidelines and an emphasis on applying common sense to the behaviour of others. These are the consequences of deliberate political choices. In order to arrest and contain the virus, considerable sacrifices have been asked of the UK public – largely without any of the scaffolding which might have supported them to make those sacrifices with the minimum possible harm. With loneliness an endemic public health problem for at least a century, many of the expectations placed on people have been emotionally unbearable, creating impossible conflicts between different kinds of survival. Without any serious acknowledgement of – or support for – these challenges, many have acted in ways which run counter to a specific public imagining of pandemic common sense, but not to their own pressing social and relational needs. Common sense is at root an invitation to judge, not to empathize or contextualize. Hiding behind a seemingly unifying language of confidence in the ability of the public to follow a particular set of standards, 'good solid British common sense' allowed shame to flourish, sowing division and dissent, and eroding the health of relationships and communities at a time where they were profoundly necessary.

As the following chapter explores, this is not the only instance in which a public rhetoric of positivity has been inextricably tangled with shame and the impulse to save face. As the government's doomed exercise in mass testing, 'Operation Moonshot', demonstrates, attempts to define public policy in proactive terms frequently resulted in the development of shame atmospheres: situations whose predication upon shame avoidance meant that shame, even when absent, remained a guiding force. As government policy was guided by efforts to save face, so too did management of the virus devolve to a politics of prestige, whose unspoken acceptance can be understood as a material consequence of common sense.

Notes

1. Hansard HC Deb 11 May 2020, vol. 676, col. 30. https://hansard.parliament.uk/commons/2020-05-11/debates/D92692B5-165B-4ACB-BC97-4C3F25D726EE/Covid-19Strategy.

2. Samuel Earle, 'Against Common Sense', *London Review of Books*, 19 July 2021. https://www.lrb.co.uk/blog/2021/july/against-common-sense.

3. Peter West, 'Why Boris Johnson Must Stop Talking about "good British common sense"', *The Conversation*, 18 June 2020, 1.10pm BST. https://theconversation.com/why-boris-johnson-must-stop-talking-about-good-british-common-sense–141008; Corsino San Miguel, 'What Is Law and What Is Guidance? The Risks of Depending on "British common sense"', *LSE Blogs*, 1 July 2020. https://blogs.lse.ac.uk/covid19/2020/07/01/what-is-law-and-what-is-guidance-the-risks-of-depending-on-british-common-sense/.

4. Roy Coleman and Beka Mullin-McCandlish, 'The Harms of State, Free-Market Common Sense and COVID–19', *State Crime Journal* vol. 10:1 (2021), 170–88. https://doi.org/10.13169/statecrime.10.1.0170.

5. Earle, 'Against Common Sense'; Anna Wierzbicka, *Experience, Evidence, and Sense: The Hidden Cultural Legacy of English* (Oxford: Oxford University Press, 2010), 337.

6. Robert Holton, 'Bourdieu and Common Sense', *SubStance* vol. 26:3 (1997), 38–52, 39.

7. Earle, 'Against Common Sense'.

8. Stuart Hall and Alan O'Shea, 'Common-Sense Neoliberalism', *Soundings: A Journal of Politics and Culture* vol. 55 (2013), 8–24, 12.

9. The Independent Scientific Advisory Group for Emergencies (SAGE), 'UK Government Messaging and Its Association with Public Understanding and Adherence to COVID-19 Mitigations: Five Principles and Recommendations for a COVID Communication Reset', 13 November 2020, 3–4. https://www.independentsage.org/wp-content/uploads/2020/11/Messaging-paper-FINAL-1-1.pdf.

10. Mass Observation Archive (University of Sussex): 12 May Day Diary, 2020 [282].

11. Reut Wertheim et al., 'Hide and "Sick": Self-Concealment, Shame and Distress in the Setting of Psycho-Oncology', *Palliative and Supportive Care* vol. 16:4 (2018), 461–9. https://doi.org/10.1017/S1478951517000499.

12. Nikolas Rose et al., 'The Social Underpinnings of Mental Distress in the Time of COVID-19 – Time for Urgent Action' [version 1; peer review: 4 approved], *Wellcome Open Research* vol. 5:166 (2020). https://doi.org/10.12688/wellcomeopenres.16123.1.

13. Mass Observation Archive (University of Sussex): Replies to Spring 2020 Directive [W6724, J2891, V3773].

14. Mass Observation Archive (University of Sussex): Replies to Spring 2020 Directive [T6654].

15. Mass Observation Archive: 12 May Day Diary, 2020 [282].

16. Stanley Rosen, 'Common Sense', *The Journal of General Education* 18:2 (July 1966), 112–36, 113.

17. Mass Observation Archive (University of Sussex): Replies to Spring 2020 Directive [O7362, C3691].

18. Mass Observation Archive Spring 2020 Directive [O7362].

19. Mass Observation Archive (University of Sussex): Replies to Summer 2020 Directive [O7362].

20. Sophia Rosenfeld, *Common Sense: A Political History* (Cambridge, MA: Harvard University Press, 2011), 14–15.

21. Rosenfeld, *Common Sense,* 4–5.

22. Wierzbicka, *Experience, Evidence, and Sense*, 349.

23. Pierre Bourdieu, *Pascalian Meditations* (Cambridge: Polity Press, 1999), 67.

24. Bourdieu, *Pascalian Meditations*, 68.

25. Wierzbicka, *Experience, Evidence, and Sense,* 367; Hall and O'Shea, 'Common-sense Neoliberalism', 8.

26. Rosenfeld, *Common Sense*, 6.

27. Clifford Geertz, 'Common Sense as a Cultural System', *The Antioch Review* vol. 33:1 (Spring 1975), 5–26; Rosen, 'Common Sense', 136.

28. Brigitte Nerlich and Rusi Jaspal, 'Social Representations of "Social Distancing" in Response to COVID-19 in the UK Media', *Current Sociology* vol. 69:4 (July 2021), 566–83, 568. https://doi.org/10.1177/0011392121990030.

29. Rosen, 'Common Sense', 127.

30. Holton, 'Bourdieu and Common Sense', 41–2.

31. Catherine V. Talbot and Pam Briggs, '"Getting back to normality seems as big of a step as going into lockdown": The Impact of the COVID-19 Pandemic on

People with Early to Middle Stage Dementia', *Age and Ageing* vol. 50:3 (May 2021), 657–63, 660. https://doi.org/10.1093/ageing/afab012.

32. Talbot and Briggs, 'Getting Back to Normality Seems as Big of a Step as Going into Lockdown', 659.

33. Rosenfeld, *Common Sense*, 15.

34. Coleman and Mullin-McCandlish, 'The Harms of State', 170; Hall and O'Shea, 'Common-sense Neoliberalism', 8.

35. Holton, 'Bourdieu and Common Sense', 45.

36. Coleman and Mullin-McCandlish, 'The Harms of State'; Stephen Reicher, Susan Michie and Ann Phoenix, 'After Restriction: Why the Public Can Only Fulfill Its Responsibilities if the Government Fulfills Theirs', *BMJ Opinion*, 29 June 2021. https://blogs.bmj.com/bmj/2021/06/29/after-restriction-why-the-public-can-only-fulfill-its-responsibilities-if-the-government-fulfills-theirs/.

37. Rosen, 'Common Sense', 120.

38. Earle, 'Against Common Sense'; Coleman and Mullin-McCandlish, 'The Harms of State', 171, 175.

39. Hall and O'Shea, 'Common-sense Neoliberalism'.

40. Rosenfeld, *Common Sense*, 4–5; Coleman and Mullin-McCandlish, 'The Harms of State'.

41. Mass Observation Archive (University of Sussex): 12 May Day Diary, 2020 [415].

42. https://www.police.uk/tua/tell-us-about/c19/v8/tell-us-about-a-possible-breach-of-coronavirus-covid-19-measures/.

43. Kevin Rawlinson, '"Rule of six": Priti Patel's Neighbours Unimpressed by Her Shopping Lawbreakers', *The Guardian*, 15 September 2020, 19.27 BST. https://www.theguardian.com/politics/2020/sep/15/rule-of-six-priti-patels-neighbours-unimpressed-about-her-shopping-lawbreakers.

44. Karen Adkins, 'When Shaming Is Shameful: Double Standards in Online Shame Backlashes', *Hypatia: A Journal of Feminist Philosophy* vol. 34:1 (2019), 76–97. http://works.bepress.com/karen-adkins/6/.

45. Mass Observation Archive (University of Sussex): 2020 Diary from non-Mass Observer [53].

46. Mass Observation Archive (University of Sussex): 2020 Diary from non-Mass Observer [47]; May Day Diary, 2020 [162]; Replies to Spring 2020 Directive [G6843].

47. Mass Observation Archive (University of Sussex): 12 May Day Diary, 2020 [39].

48. Mass Observation Archive (University of Sussex): 12 May Day Diary, 2020 [52]; Replies to Summer 2020 Directive [T5672].

49. Fred Cooper, 'COVID-19 and the Loneliness Crisis', *Solitudes Past and Present*, 2 April 2020. https://solitudes.qmul.ac.uk/blog/covid-19-and-the-loneliness-crisis/.

50. Mass Observation Archive (University of Sussex): Replies to 2020 Special Directive [C7297].

51. Mass Observation Archive (University of Sussex): 12 May Day Diary, 2020 [269].

52. Mass Observation Archive (University of Sussex): Replies to Summer 2020 Directive [M3118].

CHAPTER 6
OPERATION MOONSHOT: NOTES ON SAVING FACE

9 September 2020. At his Coronavirus Press Briefing, Boris Johnson announces 'an alternative plan' to return life 'closer to normality'.[1] The plan he proposes will use 'testing to identify people who are negative – who don't have coronavirus and who are not infectious – so we can allow them to behave in a more normal way, in the knowledge they cannot infect anyone else with the virus'. 'Our plan', Johnson continues, 'this moonshot that I am describing – will require a giant, collaborative effort from government, business, public health professionals, scientists, logistics experts and many, many more'. Criticized at the time for being 'devoid of any contribution from scientists, clinicians, and public health and testing and screening experts', and 'disregarding the enormous problems with the existing testing and tracing programme', Johnson's plan will ultimately disappear from the government's agenda, relegated to the dustbin of history.[2] However, it serves as a useful reminder of the way that the UK government's rhetoric consistently encouraged expectations vastly in excess of their capacity to deliver.

In this chapter, we argue that this mismatch provided ideal conditions for a shame environment, manifested in the numerous face-saving strategies employed by the government and their defenders to avoid public rebuke and a concomitant avoidance of responsibility. In what follows, we discuss what, exactly, was meant by Operation Moonshot, the role it played in developing unrealistic expectations, the way these expectations frequently led to public calls for accountability, and the face-saving and reputation management the government developed in response.

The effort to name and promote Operation Moonshot make it a particularly apt example for examining the UK government's efforts to save face. By September 2020, there had been numerous proposals for mass testing in the form of declared daily targets. When the targets were eventually met, the government would use these successes to mock its critics, seemingly forgetting that targets were achieved weeks, even months, after the stated deadline.[3] Importantly, these red lines were not a single occurrence but a recurrent feature of government briefings.[4] Rather than acknowledge the flaws in decision-making that raised expectations, the government would frequently cover over past failures with larger, ever more ambitious testing aims: 100,000 a day, 250,000 a day, 500,000 a day and, eventually, 10,000,000 a day. Often these announcements appeared to offset the criticisms of NHS Test and Trace, the contact tracing programme led by Dido Harding until April 2021.[5] In this context, saving face emerged as a repeated strategy to offset failures to meet the lines they had set for themselves – lines, moreover, that were set in an effort to save face.

Operation Moonshot

Moonshots, writes Gemma Milne, are 'big, ambitious, expensive projects which are hard to do and – by most measures – not all that sensible; "a crazy idea" if you will'.[6] They are 'singular', 'ego-boosting' 'and, in the long run, really not all that useful'. They are also, Milne continues, often 'used as a stand-in for solving something so complicated that any reasonable proposal for change would be seen as boring, too long-term and not at all beneficial for winning in political cycles'. Johnson's moonshot, she suggests, can be interpreted in two possible ways:

> Either [Dominic] Cummings and Johnson don't realise that using the term and approach to describe their pandemic plans is old hat, naive, and destined, in its narrowness, to not work – which suggests they have no clue what they're doing. Or they know that this narrative will add to the misinformation and confusion, picking up easy excited headlines from their champions in the press – which suggests they don't care that their plan is operationally lacking if it serves the rhetorical purpose of fooling some.[7]

These are both disturbingly viable explanations. Still, a third, less 'old hat' possibility was that they were trading on the traction that moonshot has developed in policy discussions of recent years, not least the mission-oriented approach advocated by the economist Mariana Mazzucato.

For Mazzucato, missions provide innovation with direction: 'they can provide the means to focus our research, innovation and investments on solving critical problems, while also spurring growth, jobs and resulting in positive spillovers across many sectors'.[8] The moonshot was paradigmatic of this. During his 25 May 1961 'Special Message to the Congress on Urgent National Needs', John F. Kennedy famously declared, 'I believe that this nation should commit itself to achieving the goal, before this decade is out, of landing a man on the moon and returning him safely to the earth'.[9] He reaffirmed this commitment at Rice University in September 1962, stating:

> We choose to go to the Moon in this decade and do the other things, not because they are easy, but because they are hard; because that goal will serve to organize and measure the best of our energies and skills, because that challenge is one that we are willing to accept, one we are unwilling to postpone, and one we intend to win, and the others, too.[10]

For Mazzucato, this mission-oriented thinking 'galvanized one of the most innovative feats in human history', where 'cost was not the issue: the point was to get the job done'.[11] The ancillary benefits, or 'spillovers', were 'technological and organization innovations that could never have been predicted at the beginning'.[12] It demonstrates how 'wicked problems' can be solved by 'getting the public and private sectors to truly collaborate on investing in solutions, having a long-run view, and governing the process to make sure it is done in the public interest'.[13]

It is worth noting that the original moonshot was also a face-saving exercise. By 1961, the USSR had launched Sputnik and Yuri Gagarin, the first artificial satellite and first human to orbit the earth, respectively. By proposing to land a man on the moon, Kennedy was hoping to rewrite the narrative of space exploration with the United States occupying 'a position of pre-eminence'.[14] Taking exception to Mazzucato's guiding example, Diane Coyle observes that 'the moonshot was not JFK's mission at all – but rather an intermediate "target"; the wider "mission" was "beat the Russians"'.[15] The realities of both moonshots come closer than the outcomes of their rhetoric might suggest.

Both Kennedy and Johnson hoped their respective moonshots would produce a wave of nationalistic support against an external antagonist. For Kennedy, a competitive space race with the Soviets provided 'an overall image' that would, in Linda Krug's words, 'transform us from a nation of losers into a nation of winners'.[16] For Johnson, the prospect of delivering more tests 'than any other country in Europe' would ratify his support for the Leave Campaign during the Brexit Referendum in 2016 and confirm the success of his subsequent 2019 campaign, run on the slogan 'Get Brexit

Done'.[17] Less apparent in this rhetoric are those citizens that moonshots implicitly exclude. Gil Scott-Heron's acerbic spoken word poem 'Whitey on the Moon', recorded in 1970 after the moon landing, recalls the travails facing Black and poor Americans at the same time that enormous resources were poured into Kennedy's moonshot.[18] Johnson's emphasis on testing as the route to 'more normal lives' contained a comparable absence: people with underlying health conditions, whose vulnerability made even regular testing an extremely risky operation. Still, even when thought of as a face-saving exercise, Kennedy's moonshot proved remarkably successful. Working out why may help us understand why Johnson's own face-saving exercise was not.

Kennedy's speech at Rice uses 'a transcendent rhetoric' built on three strategies: 'a characterization of space as a beckoning frontier; an articulation of time that locates the endeavor within a historical moment of urgency and plausibility; and a final, cumulative strategy that invites audience members to live up to their pioneering heritage by going to the moon'.[19] Space presented an unprecedented situation for *not* pursuing the exigencies of war and international competition. Although the space race was intended to be an opportunity to 'beat the Russians', it was framed as an opportunity to transcend such petty rivalries. It offered the opportunity to save face, while claiming to transcend the dynamics which made face-saving desirable.

The historical context and conditions of the original moonshot highlight many of the problems that manifested in Johnson's imitation. Whereas the figure of a man on the moon gave people a clear and intuitively understandable target, to be achieved in a short, but not impossible, time frame, the notion that 10 million tests a day would be rolled out by early 2021, from an existing capacity of 200,000 tests a day in September, seemed both too complicated an idea and too short a period of time in which to achieve it. As implausible as a man on the moon may have appeared, it was, at least, an easily visualized image. Johnson's moonshot relied on people imagining the difference between two impossibly large numbers. As difficult as it might have been for experts to imagine a moon landing in less than ten years, Kennedy made it easy for a lay audience, who, in the fifteen years previously, had seen the emergence of penicillin, television and nuclear power, to conceive of it.[20] The successive failures of Johnson's government to meet previously set targets made it unlikely and implausible that they would achieve this much larger one.

The success of Kennedy's moonshot was predicated on the people of the United States feeling like they had a stake in the achievement, and framing a manifestly nationalist project focused on competing with another sovereign power as if it were a noble mission for the betterment of humanity.[21] Despite its material exclusions of Black and poor Americans, it was remarkably successful as a piece of rhetoric. A 1963 Gallup poll showed 69 per cent of the population supported 'either maintaining or increasing the pace of the lunar program', against 33 per cent from a poll before Kennedy's intervention.[22] By contrast, the swiftness with which the Johnson government abandoned the moonshot suggests that British people felt less confident that 10 million tests a day would seriously 'allow life to return closer to normality'.[23] If developing a collective response to Covid-19 provides a far more legitimate claim to greater human purpose than landing a man on the moon, the great irony was that Johnson's moonshot seemed simply to fit into a tendency, on the part of the UK government, to compare their own achievements with those of other nations. The face-saving exercise had failed.

Saving face

We have suggested that both moonshots turned on questions of saving face. But what is 'face', and what does it mean to save it? In his essay 'On Face-Work', Erving Goffman defines face as 'the positive social value a person effectively claims for himself by the line others assume he has taken during a particular contact'.[24] The line is understood to be the views a person expresses to others, consciously or not, through a pattern of verbal and nonverbal acts. For Goffman, people 'have', 'are in' or 'maintain face' when the line they take is internally consistent with their self-image, and is supported by the judgements and evidence of others. When information about social worth cannot be integrated with this line, a person is in 'wrong face', while a person is 'out of face' when their line is not the one expected of a particular situation. When this leads one's manner and bearing to falter, collapse and crumble, Goffman refers to the ensuing embarrassment as becoming shamefaced: 'the feeling, whether warranted or not, that he is perceived in a flustered state by others, and that he is presenting no usable line, may add further injuries to his feelings'.[25] 'To lose face', Goffman continues, 'seems to mean to be in wrong face, to be out of face, or to be shamefaced. The phrase "to save one's face" appears to refer to the process by which the person sustains an impression for others that he has not lost face'.[26] We save face when people choose to accept the line we take despite external challenges to it.

Face is fundamentally social: however much we value it personally, face 'is only on loan to [us] from society; it will be withdrawn unless [we] conduct [ourselves] in a way that is worthy of it'.[27] Face therefore has a certain fragility. It must be shored up by rules of conduct. For the self, the rule of self-respect demands that one 'abjure certain actions because they are above or beneath [them], while forcing [themselves] to perform others even though they cost [them] dearly'.[28] When treating others, the rule of considerateness demands one to 'go to certain lengths to save the feelings and the face of others present, and … do this willingly and spontaneously because of emotional identification with the others and with their feelings'.[29] Someone who fails to live up to the rule of considerateness is considered 'heartless' and someone who fails to live up to the rule of self-respect is considered 'shameless'. While maintaining face is usually 'a condition of interaction, not its objective', under certain circumstances the actions taken to make what someone is doing consistent with their 'face', or 'face-work', prioritize saving face over the explicit reason for the intervention. It is our contention that Operation Moonshot cannot simply be considered as a technoscientific plan of great ambition, but that it also had as one of its objectives the aim of maintaining and saving face.

When Matt Hancock, then Secretary of State for Health and Social Care, presented Operation Moonshot to the House of Commons on the 10th of September 2020, he found himself subjected to laughter and heckles. These arose in response to his declaration that, once the new approach to mass testing was piloted and the technology was verified, it could be 'rolled out nationwide'.[30] Although the laughter may be understood as simply a feature of the systematic impoliteness that characterizes the Commons' adversarial political discourse, Hancock's reaction made it appear something more.[31] Hancock's own response was to 'depart from his script' and rebuke 'the nay-sayers' who complained 'that we will never get testing going… They are against everything that is needed to sort this problem for this country, and they would do far better to support their constituents and get with the programme.'[32] By announcing his departure from his script and then devoting some time to 'dressing down' his opponents, Hancock marked the laughter as 'an incident', an event 'expressively incompatible' with his line, and therefore in need of a corrective process.[33] Rather than use this process to offer redress, Hancock adopted an aggressive approach to 'introduce favourable facts about himself and unfavourable facts about the others' for the sake of his audience: Conservative MPs and, we can assume, watchers of Parliamentary Live.[34] The overwhelmingly negative response, evidenced by Twitter interactions with the announcement, suggests that this approach failed. In Goffman's words, 'he is made to look foolish; he loses face'.[35]

This anecdote tells us something about Hancock's personal efforts to maintain and save face. To argue it illustrates a general government strategy, however, we need to show how 'saving face', although a particular form of interpersonal social interaction, comes to be a material factor in matters of policy, and how Hancock's particular performance of 'saving face' fits in a longer sequence of encounters that sedimented as a collective action by the UK government. In considering the way such micro-level mechanisms for avoiding embarrassment 'produce international institutions like diplomacy', Deepak Nair argues that 'face-saving enables the performance of sovereign equality on the back of status equality; fosters in-group identity and cohesion; and serves as a micro-foundation for conflict avoidance in interactions among diplomats and statesmen'.[36] Importantly, 'saving face' for Nair does not need to be linked to culturally essentialist ideas like 'shame cultures' or 'face cultures'; instead, it can be understood as a practice, arising from social interactions, 'by which actors avoid conflict and manage contention'.[37] 'Variation in face saving is explained not by essentialist group traits', he explains, 'but how power is ordered in a given social context'.[38] Different personalities representing the UK government, like Boris Johnson or Matt Hancock, had their own techniques for saving face, reflecting their personal style and different public positions. But by both resorting to face-saving, they highlight a governmental strategy for avoiding embarrassment. Their efforts were not merely personal endeavours but aimed to order power in given social contexts.

Nair's work argues that saving face can be a legitimate technique for thinking about the impact of interpersonal dynamics in larger political contexts. But can we take Hancock's face-saving to be part of a collective action by the UK government? The first hint that we can emerges when he lays claim to this collectivism more or less explicitly by using the first person plural. Mocking the inconsistencies of the Opposition, Hancock declared: 'I have heard Opposition Members complain that we will never get testing going. They are the same old voices. They opposed the 100,000 tests, and did we deliver that? Yes, we did. They say, "What about testing in care homes?" Well, we delivered the tests to care homes earlier this week.'[39] Like attacks on the Opposition, the first person plural is a standard rhetorical feature of government. Nevertheless, three features make this 'we' particularly noteworthy.

First, the 'we' clearly refers to the government, rather than, say, other, greater polities, like 'the British People', which were typically invoked in more public updates on the crisis. This suggests that the defense of 'face', offered by Hancock, is a defense of the collective face of the government. Second, the criticisms followed a general tendency in the rhetoric of the Johnson government to present ostensibly true statements that dissimulated about context. When the government promised to deliver 100,000 tests by the end of April 2020, they met the target by including mailout tests (test sent to individuals at home or in hospitals) in the count of tests already completed.[40] Likewise, when Vic Rayner, executive director of the National Care Forum, called for a so-called 'ring of steel' around care homes in April 2020, the government promised testing for all residents and staff throughout the summer.[41] In August, they backtracked, citing 'unexpected delays', and only delivered, as Hancock said, in early September.[42] As Opposition MPs were quick to point out, the government's delivery came weeks, even months after the promised deadline. Importantly, the government used the truth of delivery to dissimulate over its failure to meet its own deadlines. Third, Hancock's response demonstrates the general tendency to use comparatives and superlatives as a way of deflecting attention away from their failure to maintain their 'line'. Here, Hancock simply compared criticisms to purported performance. Boris Johnson would present much clearer examples of these strategies during his appearances at Prime Minister's Questions over the next two weeks.

On 16 September, the Deputy Leader of the UK Labour Party Angela Rayner jibed that 'the Prime Minister has put his faith in Operation Moonshot, but, meanwhile, on planet Earth, there were no NHS tests available for several high-infection areas'.[43] In his response, Johnson defends the ambition of the plan as a matter of comparative record:

> We want to get up to 500,000 tests per day by the end of October. As I have said, that is a huge, huge number. I really do pay tribute to all those who are delivering it. I know that Opposition Members like to make these international comparisons, so I will just repeat that we are testing more than any other European country.[44]

His insistence on the 'huge number' of tests sets a numerical value and makes that value a defining quality of success. It establishes a line on the matter of testing. This line, however, is intimately connected to his desire to present a favourable comparison with Europe, a concern pronounced enough that he would return to it again in response to another of Rayner's questions:

> I think that most people looking at the record of this country in delivering tests across the nation will see that that compares extremely well with any other European country. We have conducted more testing than any other European country, and that is why we are able to deliver tests and results.[45]

On 23 September, he would return to this line of defence in his ripostes to the Leader of the Opposition, Keir Starmer:

> We are not only at a record high today, testing more people than any other European country, but that, to get to the point that the right hon. and learned Gentleman raises, we are going to go up to 500,000 tests by the end of October.[46]

There are other, more salacious examples of the government insisting on their absolute success, but this particular line is useful because it introduces a tendency towards the superlative and the hyperbolic, observable across claims about Operation Moonshot.

Superlatives express the very highest degree of a quality. Hyperbole describes expressions where claims, whether superlative or not, are more extreme than the object discussed can justify.[47] Now, comparing the performance of the UK government to other countries is not, strictly speaking, a grammatical instance of the superlative, and, when the claim can be justified, neither is it hyperbolic. But their empirical validity seems secondary to their symbolic importance. We are, after all, not as interested in whether the UK government produced more tests than other countries in Europe, as we are in why telling people matters.

Commenting on the way that urban theorists use superlatives and 'firsts' to frame their work, Robert A. Beauregard noted how the tendency led to claims being extracted from their original context, while also implying 'a hierarchy of values ... that is hardly ever revealed'.[48] For Beauregard, this meant that the theoretical implications of the claims remained unaddressed. Moreover, '[t]he deployment of superlatives and "firsts" disorients the reader by blurring the distinctions among different types of texts and interpretive stances. This, in turn, weakens our ability to evaluate the texts'.[49] Beauregard was complaining about forms of 'boosterism' in academic writing, and so his comments may not appear immediately relevant. However, he usefully points to the way that boosterism directs attention to one area, while deflecting it away from another. In the immediate context, superlatives about testing replaced superlatives about the 'worst death toll in Europe'. But it also justified Brexit to those who had voted to leave the European Union in the 2016 referendum and those who had voted for the Conservative Party in the 2019 general election so they could 'Get Brexit Done'.

By making favourable comparisons with the rest of Europe, Johnson could emphasize the successes of the UK after it left the EU on the 31st of January 2020. These claims were abstracted from a context in which other comparisons – the overall death rate, hospital beds per 100,000 – presented the UK in a much poorer light. They insisted on prioritizing particular forms of performance – expense, numerical superiority – over other, potentially more important metrics. One moment the government would discuss capacity; the next, it would be tests delivered. Neither were so significant as the number being touted: frequently in the tens of thousands, hundreds of thousands or millions, the only ambition seemed to be to make these numbers grow and grow. The aim was to present the UK's response as paradigmatic and 'world-leading', even if only its own citizens would ever believe that.

There were significant substantive and material reasons for presenting Brexit as a successful policy decision. But the personal commitment to leaving the EU, made by Johnson and many of the senior figures in his government, suggests that the need for it to succeed relied in no small way on saving face. A successful Brexit was a line, in Goffman's terms, on which face might be made, maintained or lost. Performance during the pandemic provided the means of establishing that success, through direct comparison with the UK's most immediate neighbours. Therefore, to save face in the pandemic demanded a correspondent loss of face on the part of EU member nations.

There is a further reason for thinking of Operation Moonshot as reflecting a broader concern with saving face: the ease with which both Johnson and Hancock were, even when they introduced the name, attempting to distance themselves from it. Johnson presents it as 'our plan, this moonshot that I am describing'.[50] Hancock refers to it as 'so-called Operation Moonshot'.[51] In both cases, the qualification of the moonshot, either as 'this' or 'so-called', undercuts the magnitude of the allusion by making it generic, rather than singular, or suggesting it is 'just' a name.

There were good reasons for their reservations. By the time they announced it, crucial planning documents related to Operation Moonshot had already been leaked to the *British Medical Journal*. In the article that broke the story on 9 September 2020, public health experts were cited as having 'already rounded on the plans'.[52] The line that Operation Moonshot was designed to establish had already crumbled. Johnson and Hancock's efforts to dismiss the name as comparatively insignificant seems part of a general effort to restate the line in the numbers of tests, rather than the grandiose posturing of the moonshot itself.

Shame avoidance

According to Goffman, saving face means to avoid losing face or becoming shamefaced. In other words, saving face is, in part, a tactic developed to avoid shame and favourably manage one's reputation. In our introduction, we argued that shame avoidance plays a crucial role in creating shame dynamics, even when no direct shame response seems to be in evidence. People will go to extraordinary lengths to avoid feeling shame and to avoid shameful exposure.[53] Ironically, boosterism, even as it appears at first to present opportunities for shame's opposite, pride, creates greater risk of shame, especially if and when the claims it makes are proven to be overblown or unrealistic.

In the UK government's case, this seems to have led to a form of 'gambler's ruin', where, in a bid to overcome the shame and reputation damage of prior bad claims, the government made successive bids to more and more impressive targets. This strategy may be explained by two needs. There was a short-term need to displace unfavourable superlatives about high numbers of excess deaths with more favourable superlatives about high numbers of daily tests. There was also a longer-term need to portray Brexit as the 'right' decision, by comparing the performance of EU countries unfavourably to that of the UK. Certainly, the government, as a whole, had a shared interest in responding to both these needs. In this regard, more abstract considerations like reputation, status and culture do have some traction in trying to explain why they went to such lengths to avoid losing face, even when this strategy was almost certain to come back to haunt them (the clearest example being the line the government took in defending Dominic Cummings's ill-fated trips to Durham and Barnard Castle).

Still, what became policy often seemed to be galvanized by the social dynamics of certain high-profile individuals, when called upon by the

Opposition, the press or the country to defend their line. The easiest analytic move would be to use shame avoidance to explain certain declarations as made 'on the hoof', or in response to challenges to the line, combine that with the individual's official standing, and claim that the need to turn the former into actual policy developed from the influence of the latter. Rather than approach it via this psychologizing route, which is largely circumstantial, evidence from Mass Observation demonstrates that members of the public thought the policies were attempts to hold a line and that, as attempts, they had failed.

Consider, from the 2020 Spring Directive, how one retired local government officer castigates the line taken by the government:

> Further the government have lied – not spoken in error, but actually lied – about how well things were going. Statements were made that our systems were world-beating when they were not; that we were testing x number of people a day when we were doing less than half that, etc. I know of no-one who is a medical scientist or a senior doctor who is not appalled and ashamed of this. Even radiographers have been reporting that they are fed up of seeing scans where the virus is all over lungs when the patient had received a false negative test result (they are c. 30% false negative). The government failed to shield and protect the most at risk (the old, those in care homes, those with serious medical problems) though they kept stating they were doing so. I am ashamed of being British now, whereas I was brought up to be proud. We may have 'saved the NHS' but we have not saved countless thousands of lives which would otherwise not have happened, and that was the fault of the government.[54]

This rich account illustrates a number of key themes that emerge in responses selected for their direct engagement with shame. Respondents repeatedly raised their own feelings of shame about being British, complained that the behaviour of the government was shameful and pointed out inconsistencies between what was said and what was done. These concerns obviously coincide in important ways. The mismatch between the statements and the truth create a 'shameful' failure to maintain the line. For some respondents, this made them 'ashamed of being British'. For others, it provoked them to call the government's decision-making 'shambolic, incompetent and shameful'.[55] We might think of the tendency to assign shame, whether to the self or to the government, as an unanswered call: an attempt to fill in the gap where some recognition of failure was felt to be needed, but remained lacking. By avoiding an honest and truthful admission of the facts, the government in effect created a shame vacuum, into which such accusations were hurled as a last ditch effort to assign blame somewhere.

People recognized that these efforts to ascribe shame were risky. Although certain figures emerged as particularly shame worthy – Boris Johnson, Dominic Cummings and Matt Hancock – this was coupled with the realization that they could not be held solely responsible. As another Mass Observation respondent put it,

> I have developed a particular disdain for Matt Hancock, which I sense I share with quite a lot of people. I've really resented his reprimanding tone which he's maintained consistently throughout the crisis, from criticising members of the public for not following social distancing measures when it was unclear both as to what the measures actually were and whether people were truly disregarding them, to attempting to scapegoat footballers. His tough language appears as nothing more than a front to cover how woefully inept he is in his role, but I hope he doesn't become the sole scapegoat, if and when proper scrutiny is placed on the government's handling of the crisis.[56]

On the one hand, Matt Hancock's reprimanding tone, referred to earlier in the chapter, appears to be 'a front' (a 'line') to disguise his inadequacies. On the other, this personal disdain risks occluding the blame that needs to be placed on the whole government. Whether or not the behaviour of the UK government, or certain individuals representing it, was or wasn't shameful, these accounts demonstrate that collective strategies of establishing or maintaining the line were taken by their intended audience to be shameful, even when their content seemingly had nothing to do with shame or shaming. In retrospect, the decisions of the government demonstrate a structural tendency towards shame avoidance, irrespective of the actual feelings of the individuals involved. Importantly, structural shame avoidance emerges out of the collective behaviour of these individuals, as a succession of face-saving efforts that were seen and judged by the general public. For this reason, we argue that a shame dynamic pervaded even those areas where shame seemed least applicable: the provision of mass testing that culminated in Operation Moonshot.

Operation Moonshot was not a resounding success. Although the government managed to increase its testing capacity to over 500,000 tests a day by 1st November, this wasn't the number they were 'getting' a day: just over 270,000 PCR tests were conducted.[57] To date, testing capacity has never risen above a million, while the total number of tests conducted (including lateral flow tests) reached its peak on 21 March 2021: 1,893,830.[58] Impressive numbers, of course, but nowhere near the promised 10 million. If anything, however, we have argued in this chapter that to focus on the numbers misses the point of what they were harnessed to do: to establish a line that could divert attention away from more serious, shame-worthy failures, while emphasizing the success of the UK post-Brexit. Taken as a line, Operation Moonshot, and the testing claims that preceded it, seemed to offer ample opportunities for the government to save face. However, continued failures to match the claims made with tangible results turned these bids for face maintenance into further opportunities for shame and shaming. This is reflected to some extent in the increasing belligerence with which senior government figures responded to perceived challenges of their policy. But it is perhaps most evident in the ways that the public, reflecting on the mismatch between what was promised and what was delivered, ended up turning to shame to articulate their unhappiness with the national response. Although not immediately recognizable through any manifestations of shaming practice or stigma, shame clearly played a shaping force in the government's decisions to maintain and save face.

Notes

1. Boris Johnson, 'Prime Minister's Statement on Coronavirus (COVID-19): 9 September 2020', *Prime Minister's Office, No. 10 Downing Street*. https://www. gov.uk/government/speeches/pm-press-conference-statement-9-september–2020.

2. Gareth Iacobucci and Rebecca Coombes, 'Covid-19: Government Plans to Spend £100bn on Expanding Testing to 10 Million a Day', *BMJ* vol. 370 (2020), m3520. http://dx.doi.org/10.1136/bmj.m3520.

3. For instance, Matt Hancock in the House of Commons. Hansard HC Deb 10 September 2020, vol 679, col 792. https://hansard.parliament.uk/ Commons/2020-09-10/debates/9916644B-878C-458C-A582-BA2020FC2E62/ Covid-19Update.

4. Boris Johnson would repeatedly attack Keir Starmer, Leader of the Opposition, for criticizing the government's approach.

5. Paul Waugh, 'The Covid Report Lays Bare Test and Trace Failings – Dido Harding's Mistakes Won't Be Forgotten', *iNews*, 12 October 2021. https://inews. co.uk/opinion/covid-report-test-and-trace-failings-dido-hardings-mistakes-wont-forgotten–1245616.

6. Gemma Milne, 'This "moonshot" Hype Only Illustrates No 10's Obsession with Tech Hyperbole', *The Guardian*, 15 September 2020. https://www.theguardian.com/commentisfree/2020/sep/15/moonshot-no-10-tech-hyperbole.

7. Milne, 'This "moonshot" hype'.

8. Mariana Mazzucato, *Mission-Oriented Research & Innovation in the European Union* (Luxembourg: Publications Office of the European Union, 2018), 4.

9. John F. Kennedy, 'Special Message to the Congress on Urgent National Needs', *John F. Kennedy Presidential Library*, 25 May 1961. https://www.jfklibrary.org/archives/other-resources/john-f-kennedy-speeches/united-states-congress-special-message–19610525.

10. Papers of John F. Kennedy. Presidential Papers. President's Office Files. Speech Files. Address at Rice University, Houston, Texas, 12 September 1962, 3.

11. Mariana Mazzucato, *Mission Economy: A Moonshot Guide to Changing Capitalism* (London: Allen Lane, 2021), 3, 4.

12. Mazzucato, *Mission Economy*, 4.

13. Mazzucato, *Mission Economy*, 5.

14. Kennedy, 'Address at Rice University', 7.

15. Diane Coyle, 'Dark Side of the Moonshot: Can the State Really Fix Our Broken Capitalism?', *Prospect Magazine*, 26 January 2021. https://www.prospectmagazine.co.uk/arts-and-books/mission-economy-capitalism-government-moonshot.

16. Linda T. Krug, *Presidential Perspectives on Space Exploration: Guiding Metaphors from Eisenhower to Bush* (New York: Praeger, 1991), 3.

17. Johnson, PM Statement: '9 September'.

18. Gil Scott-Heron, 'Whitey on the Moon', *Small Talk at 125th and Lenox* (Flying Dutchman/RCA, 1970). Spoken word.

19. John W. Jordan, 'Kennedy's Romantic Moon and Its Rhetorical Legacy for Space Exploration', *Rhetoric and Public Affairs* vol. 6:2 (2003), 210.

20. Jordan, 'Kennedy's Romantic Moon', 219.

21. Jordan, 'Kennedy's Romantic Moon', 211.

22. Mark E. Byrnes, *Politics and Space: Image Making by NASA* (Westport, CT: Praeger, 1994), 39–40.

23. Johnson, PM Statement: '9 September'.

24. Erving Goffman, 'On Face-Work: An Analysis of Ritual Elements in Social Interaction', On *Psychiatry* vol. 18 (1955), 213.

25. Goffman, 'On Face-Work', 214.

26. Goffman, 'On Face-Work', 215.

27. Goffman, 'On Face-Work', 215.

28. Goffman, 'On Face-Work', 215.

29. Goffman, 'On Face-Work', 215.

30. Hansard HC Deb 10 September, col 792.

31. Sandra Harris, 'Being Politically Impolite, Extending Politeness Theory to Adversarial Political Discourse', *Discourse & Society* vol. 12:4 (2001), 451–72.

32. Hansard 10 September, cols 792–3.

33. Goffman, 'On Face-Work', 222.

34. Goffman, 'On Face-Work', 222.

35. Goffman, 'On Face-Work', 222.

36. Deepak Nair, 'Saving Face in Diplomacy: A Political Sociology of Face-to-face Interactions in the Association of Southeast Asian Nations', *European Journal of International Relations* vol. 25:3 (2019), 673–4. https://doi.org/10.1177/1354066118822117.

37. Nair, 'Saving Face', in diplomacy 679.

38. Nair, 'Saving Face', in diplomacy 679.

39. Hansard 10 September, col 793.

40. Nick Carding, 'Government Counts Mailouts to Hit 100,000 Testing Target', *Health Services Journal*, 1 May 2020. https://www.hsj.co.uk/quality-and-performance/government-counts-mailouts-to-hit-100000-testing-target/7027544.article.

41. Vic Rayner, 'Ring of Steel Needed to Support Care Homes as Deaths Double in a Week', *National Care Forum*, Press Release 18 April 2020. https://www.nationalcareforum.org.uk/draft/ring-of-steel-needed-to-support-care-homes-as-deaths-double-in-a-week/.

42. Enda Brady, 'Coronavirus: Testing for COVID-19 in Care Homes Delayed Until September', *Sky News*, 2 August 2020. https://news.sky.com/story/coronavirus-testing-for-covid-19-in-care-homes-delayed-until-september–12041099.

43. Hansard HC Deb 16 September 2020, vol. 680, col. 304. https://hansard.parliament.uk/Commons/2020-09-16/debates/21E9A3A1-75C6-428F-88B8-6EDEA2A1CD36/PrimeMinister.

44. Hansard, '16 September', col 304.

45. Hansard, '16 September', col 304.

46. Hansard HC Deb 23 September 2020, vol. 680. https://hansard.parliament.uk/Commons/2020-09-23/debates/D05F8C95-1184-4E36-9737-27042B47E331/PrimeMinister.

47. Christian Burgers, Britta C. Brugman, Kiki Y. Renardel de Lavalette and Gerard J. Steen, 'HIP: A Method for Linguistic Hyperbole Identification in Discourse', *Metaphor and Symbol* vol. 31:3 (2016), 166.

48. Robert A. Beauregard, 'City of Superlatives', *City & Community* vol. 2:3 (2003), 188. https://doi.org/10.1111/1540-6040.00049.

49. Beauregard, 'City of Superlatives', 189.

50. Johnson, PM Statement: '9 September'.

51. Hansard, '10 September', col 793.

52. Iacobucci and Coombes, 'Covid-19'.

53. See, for instance, Martha Nussbaum, *Hiding from Humanity: Disgust, Shame, and the Law* (Princeton: Princeton University Press, 2004), 219.

54. Mass Observation Archive (University of Sussex): Replies to Spring 2020 Directive [Q7053].

55. Mass Observation Archive (University of Sussex): Replies to Spring 2020 Directive [A7053, W6724].

56. Mass Observation Archive (University of Sussex): Replies to 2020 Special Directive [O7365].

57. 'Testing in the United Kingdom', *Coronavirus (COVID-19) in the UK*, Accessed: 28 February 2022. https://coronavirus.data.gov.uk/details/testing.

58. 'Testing in United Kingdom'.

CONCLUSION: BEYOND PLAGUE ISLAND

In the closing weeks of 2020, an article in *The New York Times* christened Britain 'Plague Island'.[1] As the then-called 'Kent variant', a more transmissible strain of the novel coronavirus, spread rapidly through the UK, other countries swiftly closed their borders to UK travellers. Just days before officially breaking its ties with the EU, the UK was left out in the cold, with escalating rates of infection, hospitalization and death at a moment where many other countries were enjoying a comparative respite. Recalling the well-worn trope of the isolated, mysterious and deadly island in literature and film, the term 'Plague Island' went beyond an obvious commentary on pandemic management and fortune, simultaneously casting the UK as parochial and small.[2] 'Plague Island' was taken up with enthusiasm in online discourses on the failings of the Johnson government and the difficulties and disappointments of living in the UK during a pandemic, entering a lexicon (including 'Brexit Island' and 'Normal Island') which derided national exceptionalism, usually in the process of drawing attention to something bizarre or unsavoury in the happenings of the day.[3] The phrase became a means of shaming the UK, frequently from within, suggesting an inability to contain and control the virus, an incompetent and blinkered political establishment, and a corresponding and deserved contempt on the world stage. For the UK, 2020 had been a year of shame.

Closely aligned with critiques of Brexit, charges of narrow-minded parochialism also came to define counternarratives on public shaming. With over 4.5 million views at the time of writing, a short, self-shot, satirical video, 'your aunt at the NHS clap', was posted on Twitter by the comedian Will Hislop on 7 May 2020.[4] Wearing an exaggerated and sanctimonious expression, 'your aunt' names and shames households on her street for non-attendance, while clapping vigorously to the sound of banging pans. Lines such as 'number 3 ... couldn't make it? HATES NURSES', and 'number 10 ... hasn't clapped since March ... oh is she ill? Not much of a journey to the doorstep ...' cast the 'aunt' as the villain of the piece, for precisely the reason that she is eager to sow shame wherever she can. Her lack of surprise that one neighbour is missing – 'doesn't wear a poppy either' – places the aunt in a longer story of surveillance and shame, while rooting Clap for Carers in close proximity to another collective national ritual, one it can also be difficult to opt out of without losing face.[5] Before the situation deteriorates into a verbal spar with a neighbour over hypocrisy and the mutual breaking of lockdown regulations, Hislop includes a brief shot of himself, as 'your aunt', clapping with a different expression – ecstatic, even transported. The pandemic, and the opportunity for status-affirming and shaming rituals it afforded, had unlocked a particular kind of animus; this, as the framing of the video suggests, should itself be a source of shame for those who give themselves up to it.

Hislop's video constructed a particular kind of character, the self-righteous arbiter of community standards, whose habits and prejudices had been amplified and given free rein. While his intention may have been to instruct – through caricature – on the ugliness of shaming, he took sight (along with more 'serious' critics of public shaming, such as D. T. Max) at a particular iteration of shame, the surface eruptions of social judgement and blame which can be clearly identified and have been widely condemned.[6] Our account takes these visible instances of public shaming as our point of departure, rooting them in deeper systems and histories and exploring the contours of shame in scenes and situations where it may not be so quickly apparent. In this book, we have drawn from a range of literatures and theories about shame from a variety of disciplines, exploring shame's personal, social, political and institutional dimensions. Through synthesizing a range of approaches to shame, our aim has been to make coherent the idea of using a 'shame lens': a novel way of understanding how the affective forces associated with negative self-conscious emotions operate across a variety of spheres and have far-reaching, and often negative, effects. These effects, we have argued, are often diminished, overlooked or ignored. Hence, overall, the book has been concerned with using a 'shame lens' to make salient a range of personal emotional experiences, along with expressions and experiences of social and political power. Focusing on three 'types' of shame, we have explored in our various case studies (1) the explicit use of shame and shaming, (2) the implicit creation of shame and shaming as a by-product of other policies and practices and (3) shame avoidance as a means for reputation management, or 'saving face'.

Covid-19 and Shame has revolved around six distinct (but related) chapters. Some of the case studies we describe are ongoing, but others are more or less temporally fixed in 2020. Alongside our analysis of recent events, the intention of the book is to demonstrate how conditions and circumstances which may seem to have little or nothing to do with shame can be decisive factors in allowing it to occur. Hannah Farrimond's work on 'stigma mutation' has explored how 'stigma emerges, mutates, and changes in response to contexts'; similar processes can be discerned in the ways that patterns of shame shift and alter, but our contention that the political and cultural environment of the UK in 2020 was primed for shame allows for a different understanding.[7]

The themes we address, therefore, have already given rise to fresh sites of shame. In Chapter 1, 'Covidiots!: The language of pandemic shaming', we argue that new kinds of pandemic language helped foster an individualized accountability for public health noncompliance, contributing to a broader atmosphere of surveillance and shame. In January 2021, the UK government's 'Can you look them in the eyes?' campaign made use of a literal shaming gaze to encourage behavioural change. Taking the form of a series of high-resolution photographs of people looking straight to camera, wearing oxygen masks over exhausted or frightened expressions, the accompanying text offered a variation on 'look him in the eyes and tell him…': 'look him in the eyes and tell him you always keep a safe distance'; 'look him in the eyes and tell him the risk isn't real'; 'look her in the eyes and tell her you never bend the rules'.[8] The observer is implicated directly in the suffering of the person in the image; the text conjures an imaginary scenario in which they are being called to account by somebody whose life they have personally endangered. Commanded to look them in the eyes, the observer cannot help but be challenged by the message, no matter how exemplary their behaviour. Under this direct, intense and profoundly personal scrutiny, we are all covidiots; each complicit, each culpable and each worthy of shame.

In Chapter 2, 'Super-spreaders: Shaming healthcare professionals', we explore the specific shaming of healthcare workers, whether for supposedly spreading the virus or for seeming to fall short of impossibly high, militarized standards of national sacrifice. As we argued in *The Lancet* in 2021, instances of online shaming against healthcare professionals shifted in focus across the course of the pandemic.[9] As it became less plausible to think of hospitals and GP practices as particular sites of infection (i.e., as community transmission was generally accepted to be the primary vector for the virus), doctors and nurses were increasingly attacked for spreading misinformation, not Covid-19. Shortly before an appearance on the BBC's current affairs and politics programme, *Question Time*, in January 2021, the palliative care doctor and writer Rachel Clarke tweeted the day's number of Covid deaths, swiftly followed by this pre-emptive message: 'And before the deluge of abuse begins, don't bother. I am seeing these poor human beings in their final days, hours and moments of life. I am seeing it – day after day after day – and it's utterly, horribly heartbreaking.'[10] Although not always without its problems, a strain of medical activism drawing public attention to overwhelmed hospitals and exhausted staff was met with shaming, harassment and threats from Covid-19 sceptics and conspiracy theorists who continued to allege that the virus was a hoax and that doctors were party to a grand-scale deception to fool or mislead the public. From being shamed as super-spreaders (in a malign inversion of their healing role), healthcare workers were shamed as bearing false witness when they sought to show an unpalatable truth.

In Chapter 3, 'Coughing while Asian: Shame and racialized bodies', we consider shame as a component of racist rhetoric and violence, trace lineages of shaming and stigmatization in the ways that neighbourhoods with racialized communities were designated as viral 'hotspots', and unpick the role of shame in the long-standing health inequalities which framed disparities in morbidity and mortality rates. Key to each of these forms of racial shaming is an overt or implicit distinction between a white 'native' body politic and racialized outsiders, who, at one end of the spectrum, are directly responsible for bringing dirt and disease and, at the other, do not know how to behave in ways that keep themselves – and white citizens – safe. While an outpouring of racist hatred and abuse at individuals assumed to be Chinese has largely subsided, the mythos of a healthy Western country under siege from foreign diseases continues to enjoy considerable traction. Across the political spectrum, public health is often conflated with policing borders: from the ongoing actions of the UK government through the Labour Party's criticisms that the government has not gone far enough, to perspectives otherwise sensitive to the structural violence that borders impose.[11] For example, on 14 December 2021, the 'NHS staff grassroots campaign', NHS Workers Say No!, tweeted an open letter to the Conservative Party, expressing – among other things – the shattered hope that the government 'would learn from previous mistakes and ensure variants from overseas wouldn't be able to enter our tiny little isolated island'.[12] The global politics of which countries get 'red-listed', and on what grounds, follow deep hierarchical fissures which reflect the ongoing, bitter legacies of colonialism.[13] With new variants most likely to emerge in places where viral transmission is highest, it is notable that much of the world has its ability to vaccinate and protect citizens significantly compromised by the past and present actions of wealthy Western states. Without confronting the global harms perpetrated by our 'tiny little isolated island', a shaming imaginary of foreign contamination will continue to have devastating repercussions.

In Chapter 4, 'I was too fat!: Boris Johnson and the fat panic', we address the consequences of individualized responsibility for obesity in public health campaigns, as important contexts were elided by an emphasis on 'simple swaps'. A wilful misrepresentation of the politics of eating, exercise, lifestyle and choice was accompanied by a shaming accountability to the functioning of the NHS, reigniting older narratives around people with excess weight as a selfish burden on straining health systems. As mass vaccination programmes have been rolled out, similar markers of shame have been attached to people who hesitate or abstain. Rather than paying close attention to the contexts and scaffolding (including a trusting and shameless engagement with public health messaging and communication) which enable different publics to make informed decisions about vaccination, the 'unvaccinated' have increasingly taken on the characteristics of a shamed population, culpable for the spread of the virus, for other adverse health outcomes produced by a health system under strain, for lingering public health restrictions to everyday life and for their own suffering. Just as messaging which heaps 'shame on blame' actively makes people less likely to engage with public health initiatives on obesity, shame over vaccination has harmed both recipients and their likelihood of vaccine uptake, representing an unnecessary barrier to healthy choices where many exist already.[14] With vaccination rates lower among people with pre-pandemic experiences of structural abandonment and shaming, and often a justified mistrust of political and medical systems, vaccine shame has to be understood as a problem of health inequalities more broadly, with considerable potential to heighten and exacerbate entrenched processes of disparity and discrimination.

In other instances, political decisions, rhetoric and processes which contributed to an atmosphere of shame recurred almost cyclically, rehearsing scenarios which are so similar as to be practically identical. In Chapter 5, 'Good solid British common sense: Shame and surveillance in everyday life', we argued that the UK government's emphasis on common sense held members of the public accountable for the pandemic in ways that encouraged deeply damaging patterns of judgement, shame and surveillance. Unable to provide an intrinsically useful or agreed-upon code for effective public health or good pandemic citizenship, appeals to common sense served a cynical political purpose. They eroded trust in scientific expertise, flattered people who like to think that they have it, and created a shamed out-group – comparable to, and overlapping with, the 'covidiots' – who were rendered responsible both for poor health outcomes and for any restrictions to everyday life the government might have reluctantly been forced to institute in the future. Accompanying broader changes in guidance from 'stay home' to 'stay alert' in the spring of 2020, narratives on common sense dwindled conspicuously in the autumn and winter, as politically intolerable rates of infection and death forced the government to return to a more paternalistic approach. For a while at least, common sense and common health seemed irreconcilable, before the gains made by mass vaccination allowed the discourse to resurface. Thus, on 6 July 2021, the health secretary, Sajid Javid, announced that the UK had entered a 'new chapter [of the Covid-19 pandemic] based on the foundations of personal responsibility and common sense'.[15] Characteristically, Javid's positioning of common sense in close proximity to 'personal responsibility' closed the circuit between the idea and logics of free-market neoliberalism, confirming critiques of Johnson's rhetoric the year before.[16]

Finally, Chapter 6, 'Operation Moonshot: Notes on saving face', explores how attempts at shame-avoidance on international and domestic political stages resulted in hyperbolic and impossible claims over a supposedly 'world-beating' capacity for mass testing, with billions of pounds diverted to a largely unsuccessful attempt at saving face over superlative numbers of Covid-19 deaths. While some of the scenes of shame discussed in this book resulted from government attempts to deflect attention from potentially shameful actions and omissions, this instance represented a means of averting shame by attempting to foster national pride. In December 2021, as the Omicron variant of Covid-19 swept through the UK, and the government's disdain for their own regulations resulted in a long-running and damaging scandal over a Christmas party at 10 Downing Street in December 2020, Johnson and Javid were enthusiastically pushing 'a new national mission: a race between the virus and the vaccine to get as many people protected as soon as possible'.[17] Echoing the absurd overpromising of Operation Moonshot, as well as the subsequent fudging of figures and language to make it seem as though targets had in fact been met, Johnson stated on record that 'everyone eligible aged eighteen and over in England will have the chance to get their booster before the New Year'. As NHS England quickly clarified that those in question would have the chance to book – but not, crucially, to receive – their booster, a government spokesperson noted that 'we believe that those aren't in contradiction.'[18] Without indulging in a semantic analysis of the word 'get', it seems fair to argue that many viewers would have interpreted Johnson's statement as a promise that they could have their booster injection in their arms, not their diaries, before the close of 2021.

Towards shame-sensitive public health

Taken together, the six chapters of this book explore scenes and experiences of pandemic shame with long historical contexts and complex legacies and repercussions. As a politically entangled and inflected emotion, shame easily attaches to groups and individuals with histories of marginalization and exclusion. Shame can be cumulative, with sufferers becoming shame-prone, and more likely to feel the adverse effects of shame in the future. Shame is also an important component of the lived experience of health problems and inequalities, and has a self-perpetuating relationship with poor relational health. For many, shame over viral transmission or poor pandemic citizenship may have been something painfully new; for others, prior encounters with shame framed and conditioned the ways that pandemic shame could be experienced and felt. In either case, the deep or shallow marks left by shame work against vital determinants of health.[19] They compromise positive and protective feelings of relational embeddedness, and erode trust in social and medical systems. They contribute to feelings of isolation and alienation, whether incremental or acute; in extreme cases, they can ignite a lifelong relationship with shame which severely curtails the possibility for security, connection or social and political engagement. Already undergoing painful processes of collective trauma and grief, populations unnecessarily subjected to shame are populations with a weakened capacity to stay well.[20] In attaching most forcefully to groups who have long experiences of exclusion, pandemic shame should also be considered as a significant vector for, and component of, entrenched health inequalities in the UK and beyond.

Part of a knowing structural inattention to the social and emotional dimensions of the pandemic has been a wilful ignorance of shame; a substantial body of evidence, particularly around HIV, could have formed the basis for sustained measures to pre-empt and disrupt processes of shaming and othering which could have been predicted to emerge in pandemic conditions.[21] A counter-history of the UK government's response to Covid-19, in which shame was confronted and mitigated, not stoked and indulged, would be a history with a host of better outcomes. Across this book, we have shown how public health initiatives which lean on shame as an emotional driver land in unforeseen and damaging ways, and trade short-term behavioural changes for long and intractable problems; when, indeed, they work at all. Shame, we contend, should never be a desired or tolerated outcome in public health.

Shame can probably never be fully eliminated from matters of illness, suffering and disease, but principles for shame-sensitive practice developed by Dolezal and Gibson for human services (e.g., medical, police and social work) offer a useful starting point for what we might term shame-sensitive public health.[22] For Dolezal and Gibson, shame should be *acknowledged*, through individual and organizational understandings of shame, attention to diversity in shame experiences and shame recognition in personal encounters; *avoided*, through an ethical commitment to rejecting shaming behaviour on an individual and collective basis, and to the frequent evaluation of practice; and *addressed*, by engaging with individual experiences of shame, fostering shame resilience and sustained opposition to the systemic causes and contexts that frame and produce the problem.[23] Not all these principles are adaptable to public health settings, particularly where they concern individual casework; translated and expanded, however, they offer a route to public health work with a critical and expansive handle on shame.

None of these measures have been seriously beyond the capability of policymakers in the past two years. As authors and academics, we tread a difficult line; we argue against the overt, tacit or accidental production of shame in public health, demonstrate its harms and attempt to set out an alternative. At the same time, we have to acknowledge that the case studies we explore have not always been a simple matter of people in positions of influence lacking the right information or evidence or having not yet been persuaded. Our uncomfortable conclusion is that shame has played a part in the pandemic which, rather than being detrimental to everyone, has been useful to some at the direct expense of the most marginalized and vulnerable. It has been, in short, a wilful political decision to create shame or to allow it to spread, a means of shifting focus away from bad governance; whether through immediate failings within the parameters of the pandemic or through long-term failings in moral leadership (such as continuing to preside over profound health inequalities predicated on racialization). A government routinely described as 'shameless' has expected us to feel their shame for them.[24] However roundly they are condemned, the deeper problem lies with the logics they perpetuate; shame is intrinsic to neoliberal languages of personal accountability, to the privatization of the political that entails. Addressing shame in public health contexts has to be part of a broader conversation about where responsibility for health is situated and whose interests that serves.

Notes

1. Benjamin Mueller and Isabella Kwai, 'For U.K., an Early Taste of Brexit as Borders Are Sealed', *The New York Times*, 21 December 2020. https://www.nytimes.com/2020/12/21/world/europe/brexit-covid-uk.html.

2. Ian Kinane, *Theorising Literary Islands: The Island Trope in Contemporary Robinsonade Narratives* (London and New York: Rowman & Littlefield International, 2016).

3. Paul Walsh, 'Trapped on Brexit Island', *Open Democracy*, 30 August 2018. https://www.opendemocracy.net/en/transformation/trapped-on-brexit-island/; Des Fitzgerald, 'Normal Island: COVID-19, Border Control, and Viral Nationalism in UK Public Health Discourse', *Sociological Research Online* (November 2021). https://doi.org/10.1177/13607804211049464.

4. Will Hislop, 'Your Aunt at the NHS Clap #nhsclap', Twitter, 7.05 pm, 7 May 2020. https://twitter.com/willdhislop/status/1258457955189641224?lang=en.

5. John Kelly, 'A Critical Discourse Analysis of Military-Related Remembrance Rhetoric in UK Sport: Communicating Consent for British Militarism', *Communication & Sport* (November 2020). https://doi.org/10.1177/2167479520971776.

6. D. T. Max, 'The Public Shaming Pandemic', *The New Yorker*, 28 September 2020. https://www.newyorker.com/magazine/2020/09/28/the-public-shaming-pandemic.

7. Hannah Farrimond, 'Stigma Mutation: Tracking Lineage, Variation and Strength in Emerging COVID-19 Stigma', *Sociological Research Online* (August 2021), 3. https://doi.org/10.1177/13607804211031580.

8. Ray Earwicker, 'Shame, Blame and Back Again: Policymaking in the Age of COVID', *Shame and Medicine blog*, 31 January 2022. https://shameandmedicine.org/shame-blame-and-back-again-policymaking-in-the-age-of-covid/.

9. Luna Dolezal, Arthur Rose and Fred Cooper, 'COVID-19, Online Shaming and Healthcare Professionals', *The Lancet* vol. 389 (2021), 482–83.

10. Rachel Clarke, 'And Before the Deluge of Abuse Begins, Don't Bother. I am Seeing These Poor Human Beings in Their Final Days, Hours and Moments of Life. I am Seeing It – Day after Day after Day – and It's Utterly, Horribly Heartbreaking', Twitter, 6 January 2021, 4:26 p.m. https://twitter.com/doctor_oxford/status/1346855625834303488.

11. Fitzgerald, 'Normal Island'.

12. NHS Workers Say NO!, 'Our Letter to the Whole of the Tory Party ...', Twitter, 10:50 p.m., 14 December 2021. https://twitter.com/nursesayno/status/1470889 058293501953?lang=en-GB.

13. Na'eem Jeenah, 'Omicron Reveals Racism against Africans, Once More', *Politics Today*, 14 December 2021. https://politicstoday.org/omicron-reveals-racism-against-africans-once-more/.

14. Graham Scambler, *A Sociology of Shame and Blame: Insiders versus Outsiders* (Basingstoke: Palgrave Macmillan, 2020), 79.

15. Hansard HC Deb 6 July 2021, vol. 698, col. 793. https://hansard.parliament. uk/Commons/2021-07-06/debates/E4E40565-A8A2-46F4-BFC0-DAEE0C5948B6/Covid-19Update.

16. Fred Cooper, 'Shame, "Common Sense", and COVID-19: Notes from Mass Observation', *Shame and Medicine blog*, 6 July 2021. https://shameandmedicine. org/shame-common-sense-and-covid-19-notes-from-mass-observation/.

17. Hansard HC Deb 14 December 2021, vol. 705, col. 944. https://hansard. parliament.uk/commons/2021-12-14/debates/8034393B-C568-4DE6-8695-1D63F957537E/PublicHealth.

18. Nadine Batchelor-Hunt, 'Chaos as Boris Johnson and NHS make Conflicting Promises over Booster Rollout', *Yahoo News*, 13 December 2021. https:// uk.news.yahoo.com/boris-johnson-and-nhs-give-different-advice-on-boosters-121300299.html.

19. Luna Dolezal and Barry Lyons, 'Health-Related Shame: An Affective Determinant of Health?', *Medical Humanities* vol. 43:4 (2017), 257–63. https:// doi.org/10.1136/medhum-2017-011186.

20. Shadan Hyder, 'COVID-19 and Collective Grief', *Child & Youth Services* vol. 41:3 (2020), 269–70. https://doi.org/10.1080/0145935X.2020.1834999.

21. Mark Honigsbaum, *The Pandemic Century: One Hundred Years of Panic, Hysteria and Hubris* (Cambridge, MA: Penguin, 2020).

22. Luna Dolezal and Matthew Gibson, 'Beyond a Trauma-Informed Approach and towards Shame-Sensitive Practice', *Humanities and Social Sciences Communications* 9:214 (2022), 1–10.

23. Dolezal and Gibson, 'Beyond a Trauma-Informed Approach and Towards Shame-Sensitive Practice'.

24. See for example 'The Guardian View on Boris Johnson: A PM without Shame', *The Guardian*, 31 January 2022, 19.23 GMT. https://www.theguardian.com/commentisfree/2022/jan/31/the-guardian-view-on-boris-johnson-a-pm-without-shame; Hugo Rifkind, 'What Does It Take for a Politician to Resign?', *The Times*, 4 May 2021. https://www.thetimes.co.uk/article/what-does-it-take-for-a-politician-to-resign-f3tmj70cr; Nigel Warburton, 'Why Shaming Boris Johnson for His Self-serving Antics is Unlikely to Work', *The New European*, 18 November 2021. https://www.theneweuropean.co.uk/why-boris-johnson-is-like-diogenes-of-sinope/.

INDEX

Locators followed by 'n.' indicate endnotes

Index

Index

Index